Helping Birth

YOUR GUIDE TO
PAIN RELIEF CHOICES
AND INTERVENTIONS
IN LABOUR AND CHILDBIRTH

with real stories

Designed, Typeset and Published by Bookzang 2018

First published in Great Britain 2018 by Bookzang.

ISBN-13: 978-1984249623

Back cover photo by Natalee Corby, with permission from Natalee Corby and Sarah Sheen.

Find great articles, information and support for pregnancy, labour and birth, and parenthood, go to:

www.birthzang.co.uk

Contents

Acknowledgements

Thanks to Olga and Simon Abreu who asked me to give them extra training to help educate them about all the pain relief options and common birth interventions. That workshop formed the basis for this book.

Thanks to all the Birthzang mums who shared their stories about using medical pain relief and who experienced common interventions: Andrea Smith, Anna Hutt, Anna Steel, Astrid Charles, Briget Stanley, Cassie C., Delyth Mair Edwards, Ellie Sonders, Emily Harwood, Fabienne Gray, Faye Bell, Jenn Runde, Jennifer Fox, Jo Linzinger, Kat D., Katie, Katy Meade, Kiera Hay, Laura Baker, Lisa Lisle, Louise Collins, Lucrezia Linardi, Macey Cansdale, Michaela Brown, Natalee Corby, Rachel Pollard, Roberta Windmill, Siobhan Marsh, Stefanie Cooper, Tanya Purdham.

Thanks to Fabienne Gray who tirelessly edited and proof-read the book, and coached me through the references! Thanks also to Suewan Kemp, and Francis and Celia Hayes who also checked the proofs meticuously.

Is this book for me?

When you see a book about choosing pain relief in labour and describing common interventions in labour and birth, it would be easy to assume that the agenda is to encourage and validate these choices of medical intervention in childbirth.

In fact, my agenda is more about facilitating education about labour and birth and the ways in which we can help this process if required. So anyone who is pregnant or supporting someone who is pregnant can make informed and objective choices.

In my experience as an Active Birth antenatal teacher (and, to a lesser extent through my yoga classes with pregnant and postnatal mums) I have heard time and again how women have opted for things they really know nothing about and as a result suffered unexpected consequences.

In an ideal world, we would have an hour for every midwife visit and all our possible choices, decisions and risks would be outlined in detail, well in advance, so that we could all contribute to our antenatal care.

In reality these visits are 10 minutes — and this in the UK; other countries not under a midwife-led system may not even have this. The onus is on us to understand what we are being told, what it means for our own personal circumstances and how it could impact pregnancy, labour and birth in both positive and negative ways.

The ultimate aim of this book is to ensure that women and their birth partners have a positive experience of labour and birth.

For some people this means a home birth, for others it means birthing at hospital. Some women cope easily with the sensations of labour and some find it the most difficult thing they have done in their life. Some mothers want only a natural birth with no outside help at all and some feel that intervening in the process is not only preferable but necessary to ensure they have a positive experience.

My job is not to make judgement of peoples choices in their pregnancy, labour and birth, but merely to provide them with a wealth of information to ensure those choices are made with insight, knowledge and understanding.

When people make informed choices about labour and birth, their experience is far more likely to be a positive one.

Who this book is for

This book is for people who want to get a top line overview of pain relief options and interventions but also dig into the detail.

This book is for people who know nothing about birth and people who know lots about it.

This book is for people who are having their first baby and second and third and fourth.

This book is for people who are scared of birth and are terrified by the mere idea of labour and people who feel supremely confident.

This book is for people who want a reference guide to look something up quickly and people who want to absorb every detail and read the book from cover to cover.

This book is for people who want to know more, who want to educate themselves and empower themselves and people who would rather not know anything.

In short, this book is for you.

Real life experience

One of the ways I felt was helpful to illustrate the ways choices and decisions in labour can affect your experience is by including real life stories of women who have had that experience.

Every chapter includes at least one real life story from a person who is part of the amazing Birthzang community. Some names are real and some are psudeonyms.

Many experiences involve more than one pain relief or intervention and I have placed them in the chapter that I feel is most relevant.

By including real stories, I hope to show that every birth is different and the way you experience that birth will be unique to you.

You cannot predict or control your birth, but you can decide how to react to it.

Part 1
Introduction and Context

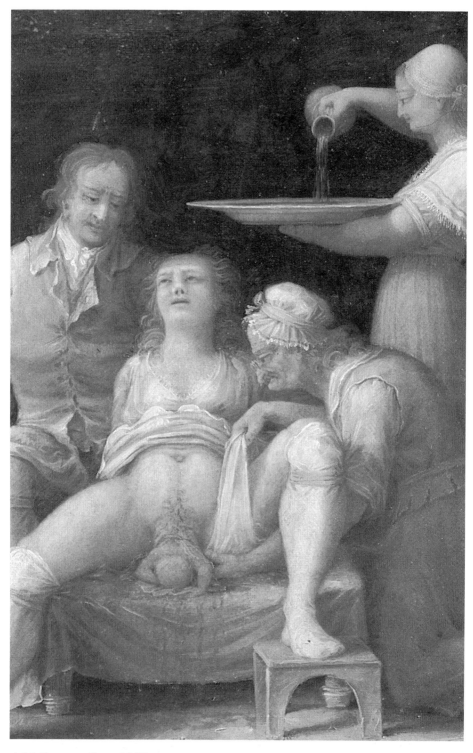

A birth scene from 1800.

Chapter 1
Introduction

Einstein – *'the only really valuable thing is intuition'*.

Most people would prefer a natural birth. When you get down to the fundamental reasons for our existence, maintaining the population has to be there at the top. Every creature procreates and there is a wonderful diversity of methods in delivering new progeny into the world.

Humans have a particularly complex way of birthing their babies. This process has evolved over millennia to ensure a beautiful symbiosis of the anatomy and physiology of mother and baby moving with each other in a carefully choreographed dance of labour and birth.

Historically, this process has been fairly successful. That said, it is a complex process with many contributing factors, some of which can cause complications putting the mother and/or baby at risk.

Maternal mortality rates[1] and infant mortality rates[2] have drastically reduced in the past 200 years. Of course, there are many changes in terms of education, understanding of the process of birth, improvements in health and welfare, better hygiene and all sorts of other sociological factors that have influenced these rates.

Ultimately, these factors result in better medical intervention and while the medicalization of birth since the 19th century has had its own set of problems, the fact remains that the improvements in pain relief for labour, and birth interventions have saved many lives.

This medicalization of birth[3] has seen the 'management' of birth taken from the hands of mothers (and experienced midwives, either qualified or not), who birthed in comfort and peace, who allowed their bodies and instincts to guide them through birth doing whatever position or movement felt right to them, into the hands of highly-educated, risk-aware obstetricians in an uncomfortable medical environment. They handed over control to someone trying to facilitate a successful birth but inadvertently had a negative impact in the labour process. This is usually by insisting the mother lay back on the bed and allow the doctor to 'deliver' the baby.

I am not the first person to resent this corruption of the natural birth process. Luckily recent thinking in the light of the ideas and teachings of such eminent childbirth experts as Sheila Kitzinger, Michel Odent, Ina May Gaskin and Janet Balaskas (who all recognized that allowing a mother to be undisturbed, in a private place and left to let her instincts guide her is the best way to facilitate a 'successful' birth) has started to swing our understanding of the best ways to redirect birthing methods back towards the more natural and ancient ways.

Many antenatal programmes enhance this understanding by teaching women to avoid lying on their backs in labour (Active Birth[4]), to practice calmness and deep breathing to help surrender to the process (Hypnobirthing[5]) and to have faith in the body's natural ability to give birth without worrying about it matching the timelines and progress by which modern birth is measured.[6]

I, myself, teach Janet Balaskas's Active Birth techniques to parents and I have found that, among my clients, many have gone on to have straightforward and natural births. Some, however, have experienced difficulties and complications meaning that they needed a bit of a helping hand.

Fortunately Active Birthing techniques are designed to allow us to embrace medical pain relief and interventions if chosen or required, and acknowledge the incredible medical advances that save lives.

Many parents don't want to even think about their births not going to plan. When they are unexpectedly faced with having to make choices and decisions about using pain relief or requiring an intervention, they are doing so without being fully informed of what they are agreeing to. Making such choices in the throes of a difficult labour is not the best time to research your options.

It is very difficult to encourage parents to find out as much as they can about birth but also not to be swamped by scary stories of birth. They need to avoid scaremongering and obsessing about what could go wrong, while ensuring that they are really educated about what is available to them should they need it.

This book is intended to educate parents about all of the pain relief options that are available to help women cope with labour and to cover the most common types of birth intervention that are encountered. This information is offered in a factual and impartial way, so that you feel fully informed about the pros and cons of each option available to you.

So, if your birth doesn't go to plan and you choose or need a helping hand, you understand fully the implications of what you are choosing.

This information is based on the UK medical system, but will not vary significantly in the US, Canada and Europe and, for that matter, the rest of the world.

How likely is it that will I need help?

While statistics will only give you one side of the story and can always be manipulated somewhat, they are nevertheless a useful benchmark to start with. Here are some statistics taken from the NHS Statistics website and Birth Choice UK,[7] an organisation that collates statistical information from hospitals across the UK to help birth professionals and women make more informed choices about birth.[8]

Statistics take time to collate and summarise and different organisations look at different data but I have done my best to make sense of it in summary.

Overall, in 2010–11, 58.2% of births in the UK had some sort of medical intervention.

We have slightly more up-to-date numbers for specific interventions and in 2016–17, 29.4% of births included an induction (including augmentation of labour), 12.7% had an assisted delivery (forceps or ventouse), and 27.8% resulted in a caesarean section (15.7% Emergency CS, 12.1% Elective CS).

In 2016–17, 60% of births required some form of pain relief (not including gas and air), showing that the likelihood of needing to be informed is quite high! While statistics on pain relief use are harder to find, it is clear that epidural rates are as high as 38.5%[9].

So, is it useful to wallow in statistics like these? Not hugely, but it paints a picture that shows that pain relief and interventions are endemic in our birth culture. That said, just because a statistic is high does not mean that it will necessarily apply to you.

Unless you have a medical condition that means you are more likely to have a medicalised birth, there is no reason why you can't have a natural birth.

Statistics give an average view but if we dig a bit deeper into them, then it is clear that just because there is a statistic that 50% do Y, that does not equate to you having a 50% chance of it happening to you.

Let's look at the statistic of 26.2% of births ending in a caesarean section.

This is the national average for the whole of England. When you look at individual hospitals you discover that this statistic varies between 15–34% depending on the hospital. So just where in the country you have your birth, the attitude and actions of the staff, and also the choices and decisions you make will all have an influence on your experience and the type of birth you might have.

Nevertheless, I still think it is *essential* to be fully informed. And the last place that you want to be informing yourself about the risks of an epidural is at hospital while deep in the throes of labour.

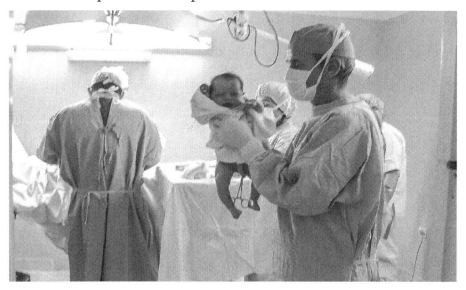

Most babies in the UK are born in a hospital or midwife-led unit.

But what will it feel like?

It's all very well learning the facts and figures about a given drug or procedure, but what can often be the most valuable resource is hearing other women's real-life stories about their experiences of using pain relief options and having interventions.

Often more than one drug or intervention happens during a birth and so it is tricky to disentangle the experience of a particular procedure in itself. However, being able to draw on the experience of others can help give you a much more real sense of how things pan out in labour, and what the decision-making process looks like when you are in the room, you are tired, and you have chosen to give your birth a helping hand.

Interspersed throughout this book are numerous stories from women in and around my network who have had a variety of types of births, with a variety of experiences – some of them very positive, some of them not so much.

These stories serve to show a picture of what happens to real people. I have had to exercise caution in selecting stories that give a true picture and yet don't fall into the category of horror stories. It would be disingenuous of me to scare women who are looking to this book as a way to learn about how we can assist in birth without feeling that there is judgement upon their decision, whether they choose an intervention, or it is thrust upon them through their personal circumstances.

I also think it is not helpful to only give rose-tinted views of beautiful births because birth is primal, it is tough, it is challenging, and yet it can be the most incredible and empowering experience of your life – intervention or not! Your attitude and the way you deal with the situation goes a long way towards shaping the experience you are going to have.

If you can arm yourself with plenty of facts about what might be on the cards, then at all times you can make informed and empowered choices and decisions, knowing that you are doing the very best for you and your baby at every step of the way.

Chapter 2
Communication, Consent and Decision-Making

Communication with birth professionals

Before we go into the details of different pain relief options and interventions, it is important to understand why we might choose this path, and how we should go about it.

The first and perhaps most important thing to consider is the people who are there to guide us through birth: midwives, obstetricians and maternity nurses. If we come into a hospital with a self-righteous attitude we are likely to clash with the people who are there to care for us. I have never met a midwife who wasn't lovely. Birth professionals often have an uncanny ability to build a strong and instant rapport with parents. We need to be careful that we don't have an 'us and them' mentality and while we may sometimes want to question their advice, and utilise our rights to make choices for our own care, this is not a personal sleight on them and their knowledge.

When we collate statistics around birth and combine them with studies around particular drugs or techniques, organisations such as NICE (National Institute for Health and Care Excellence) provide guidelines around which hospitals can structure their care plan. These guidelines often become incorporated into a hospital's policy and then, somewhere along the way, recommendations can turn into a firm policy via the language used.

For example, instead of the NICE recommendation that every woman with an uncomplicated pregnancy should be routinely *offered* an induction between 41–42 weeks of pregnancy,[10] most women are *booked in* for an induction by week 40 and it is often discussed with them much earlier.

This distinction between policy and guideline is one that is often overlooked by care providers. You are entitled to make different choices than the ones your care providers present to you and still be adhering to

NICE guidelines. Working with your care team is the best way to ensure you make the best choices for you both to achieve the care plan that you want, even if it is not strictly aligned with hospital policy.

It is so important to have the attitude of working *with* your care providers and not against them. If you are really informed about pain relief options and interventions and you are asking relevant, specific and pertinent questions, then you will ensure you have open and helpful conversations with them. In some cases, you need to be firm and stick to your knowledge and rights, but in my experience if you are informed then you work together with your birth team in such a way that you feel supported and they feel that they are being supportive. It is win–win!

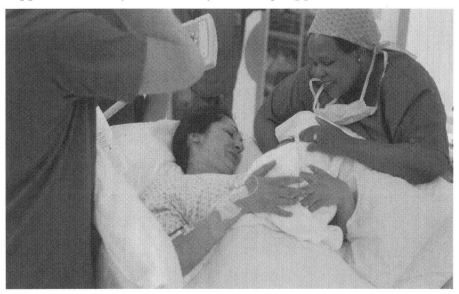

Midwives have an uncanny ability to quickly build up a rapport with parents

Informed consent and your rights

For many women, the language surrounding birth is a reflection of the way we walk into a hospital and submit our control to the professionals. We believe that the things that happen during labour and birth happen to us, that the decisions are made by the birth professionals and that they are the best people to make that decision for us.

In many cases, we refer to being 'allowed' to do something, when the truth of the matter is that it is all our *choice*.

We are wrapped up in the cultural opinion that birth is a medical event and, as we would if we had a serious medical condition such as a broken leg or appendicitis, we are quite happy to relinquish the decision-making to the doctors: they are the experts after all.

However, birth is no more a medical event than having a poo, menstruating or blinking (although does require quite a bit more effort!). All these are natural bodily processes that nature has designed to work pretty effectively. While we usually feel safer having our babies in a hospital or birthing centre, it is our choice to do so, and that choice extends to every single aspect of birth.

There is always more choice than is apparent – things are often presented as one option only, particularly with interventions. 'I am just going to give you an injection to deliver the placenta', is a good example of a birth professional assuming that a woman gives consent to a routine procedure.

In some cases, the health and wellbeing of the mother, or particularly the baby, are cited as the reason for making the decision, and in certain cases we'd be insane not to follow this advice. If your baby's heartbeat is compromised, there is no question that intervention is necessary.

Unfortunately, our risk-averse medical profession sometimes loses sight of the body's natural ability to birth a baby, especially when it comes to going into labour spontaneously, and the 'risks' to our baby for following a natural approach are often minimal.

There are always choices. Understanding the true benefits and risks of drugs and medical interventions is the only way to make the best decision for you and your baby.

Permission

Birth is something you are doing in the company of birth professionals to ensure that everyone is as safe as possible. While you may be asked, recommended or told to do certain things, you don't need permission to:

- get off the bed (even if you are on a monitor)
- go to the toilet
- eat or drink (unless you are scheduled for a general anaesthetic)
- change position
- decline a treatment
- ask for a treatment to be stopped
- change your mind.

What rights do I have?

Remember that you are not a child; you are a fully-grown consenting adult who can vote, drive and take responsibility for your life. Birth is no exception and you have a right to:

- decline treatment
- ask people to leave
- ask for different midwife
- have a home birth
- get a second opinion
- speak to the supervisor midwife or consultant midwife about any concerns.

Decision-making

So how can you make good decisions during labour?

A fantastic resource for parents is the BRAIN acronym, widely used among antenatal teachers to help assess whether or not to choose pain relief or interventions in labour. Its origins are not very clear (and if you know please get in touch!) but the earliest example I could find was birth educator Mary Nolan,[11] who mentions it in her books about teaching antenatal classes.

The BRAIN acronym stands for:

Benefits

Risks

Alternatives

Implications/Interventions

Nothing.

Let's have a deeper look at each of these questions.

B - What are the BENEFITS of this course of action?

Of course, all pain relief options and interventions come from a perspective of giving birth a helping hand and so the benefits are usually obvious. Nevertheless, it is still helpful to be really clear about all of the positive outcomes of the intervention, just to be sure you are all talking about the same thing.

R - What are the RISKS?

An obvious next step is to look at the risks of the intervention. We are referring here to the risks to the mother, and to the baby, and also a risk to the benefits of the intervention. Sometimes risks are presented in a misleading way, so make sure you ask for specific statistics for that intervention to be clear on the difference between relative and actual risk (*see* Chapter 3: Understanding Risks).

A - Are there any ALTERNATIVES?

What alternative options are there instead of taking this course of action? In some cases, it is all or nothing, but there are sometimes other paths that are just not presented as part of the picture.

I - What are the IMPLICATIONS of following this course of action? Will it make further INTERVENTIONS more likely?

This is a key part of the decision-making process as implications are rarely discussed when you are looking at interventions. We automatically balance the benefits and risks but we don't take into account what might happen as a result of the intervention. This is known in the birthing world as the 'cascade of intervention', a term coined by home birth midwife Pam England,[12] meaning that starting one type of intervention often leads to a succession of others.

This is most obviously seen in the result of the use of epidurals and also during induction of labour.

N - What if we do NOTHING and wait for an hour or two before taking action?

This is an interesting perspective and one that goes back to the simpler view of birth that patience is key and many 'complications' surrounding birth are more about birth not fitting into our measurements and guidelines (usually around time), rather than an actual problem.

Sometimes just asking for time to think about it will let you know if there is indeed time to reflect (in which case, what is the drama all about?). This is also a good delay tactic if you are feeling under pressure to make a decision that you are not ready to make.

Questions to ask

So how can you communicate this decision-making process with your care team? Asking specific questions can help you elicit some of the answers to help you make an informed choice.

- Why do you feel I need this drug/procedure?
- Am I or the baby in imminent danger?
- What are the benefits for me of this drug/procedure?
- Is this drug/procedure being offered because of routine policy, or because of my or my baby's specific circumstances?
- What are the risks for this drug/procedure?
- What alternatives are there?
- What kind of monitoring will I need?
- What would happen if I did nothing?
- Can I think about it for a few days/hours?
- Can I get a second opinion?

Just remember that it is valid to say 'yes' and 'no' and 'thanks, I am going to think about it' in answer to any question about your care.

But what if there is no time to reflect?

In some instances, there is no time to pause, reflect and ask lots of questions – this is a true emergency. You generally get a sense of this because the entire atmosphere in the room will change. Tones of voice will change, buttons will be pressed, people turn up and you will know very clearly that the time for choice has passed and this is the moment to let the experts do their thing.

However, usually in most situations there is time to reflect and consider. And so, it is always worth probing and making sure you are making the right choice for you and your baby.

Chapter 3
Understanding Risks

All medical interventions have benefits and risks. While the benefits will probably be quite obvious, the risks are not always so clear. There are often a number of things to consider:

- Side effects of intervention
- Likelihood of those side effects
- Possible complications of intervention
- Likelihood of those complications.

The side effects and possible complications are usually like a list of ingredients just as with any medication you come across. The likelihood of these effects and complications occurring is where the true risk becomes apparent and this takes us back to statistics.

As we saw from the caesarean statistic in Chapter 1, you need to look at the statistics in the context of the specific hospital you are in. Birth Choice UK has all of this information.

But we also need to start to understand relative risk and absolute risk.

Relative risk

Many times, the risk of an intervention (or of not doing the intervention, for example, having an induction to start your labour) is often couched in terms of increase of risk or relative risk.

If you are told that if you don't do an intervention then your risk of your baby coming to harm are doubled, then that is terrifying and you would automatically consent to an intervention. A good example is that women are often told that they need to induce their labour as the risk of stillbirth doubles between 40–42 weeks of pregnancy. This is obviously very scary!

Who wouldn't want to avoid doubling this risk? All we hear is 'double the risk' without considering what the *likelihood* is of it happening in the first instance.

This is the relative risk. This (negative?) outcome is twice as likely if you don't do this intervention. It is much easier to explain in terms of doubling, or halving, rather than spouting numbers at people.

Unfortunately, this can be a rather misleading way to look at risk.

Absolute risk

Absolute risk starts to dig a little deeper into the actual statistics. If we take risk of stillbirth at term then we can see that, according to NICE, there are 0.9 per 1000 births at 40 weeks, and by 42 weeks that number has gone up to 1.6 per 1000.[13]

Yes, there is a doubling of the risk but the actual risk, the absolute risk is still very tiny and also doesn't take into account known medical condition or circumstances that may affect this number.

And yet the risks associated with induction remain quite numerous and varied, both in the context of labour and birth, and also for the baby in the days and weeks after birth.[14] I will discuss this in more detail in Part 4: Induction, but suffice it to say you need to dig deep into risk to be able to fully understand what that risk means.

Chapter 4
The Physiology of Labour

While this book is primarily a discussion about the experience of using pain relief and interventions during labour and birth, it helps to have an understanding of the process of labour and the different stages it goes through. This is because certain options are only used in certain stages of labour.

The stages of labour

Labour is segmented into three distinctive stages of labour, and the first stage itself can be further segmented into three phases: latent labour, established labour and transition. They have quite distinctive characteristics so it is worth covering them separately, even though they are really considered to be one stage.

First stage - latent phase (pre-labour)

This stage is considered to commence from the first indications that labour is starting. There are many ways this can occur and some women can have mild contractions for days if not weeks before labour proper starts (hence the term pre-labour). It can be hard to distinguish the exact starting point of this stage as the start of labour can be one or a combination of: period pain, cramps, mild contractions, losing mucous plug, water breaking.

How can I tell I am in this phase?

Once you have signs that labour is starting, then you would be considered to be in this phase of Stage 1. As this phase progresses, contractions will last for around 30–60 seconds with long or erratic gaps between them. There is often no regular pattern of contractions at this stage – much like an orchestra tuning up before a concert!

What is happening in the body?

The cervix starts hard and tightly closed, and sits high and far back in the vagina. The purpose of the contractions is to push the baby's head against the cervix to soften it, move it down the vagina, thin out (efface) and start to open. By the end of the latent phase, the cervix is open to around 4cm in dilation. The baby is also changing position during the first stage of labour and will optimally start facing sideways towards the mother's right hand side and will begin to rotate to face backwards.

What is clear, and why it is considered separately, is that the latent phase is the most unpredictable part of labour. It is the body's way of warming up and finding its rhythm. It can speed up and slow down. You can be dilated with gentle contractions, or have intensive contractions with no dilation.

What marks progression is the combination of a few variables that mean contractions become more effective and start to cause dilation.

How does it feel?

The initial feelings of the first stage of labour are very subtle and you can often carry on with normal activities in the early parts of this stage.

Contractions start fairly short, mild and irregular, and become more frequent, longer in duration, and build up into a regular pattern. Generally, the signs and symptoms of labour are quite gentle and fairly erratic. There are often many minutes or even hours between early contractions and you are usually able to continue to talk during a contraction.

The intensity and pain of each contraction will increase as the labour progresses, and towards the end of the latent phase you need to start to focus on each contraction.

How long does it last?

The question of how long the latent phase of labour lasts is an impossible one to answer categorically. We work on averages but for every person who matches this average, there are some who have much shorter labours and some who have much longer ones. The erratic nature of the latent phase is why it is not counted towards labour length in your records, and why you are not admitted to hospital until you have reached the established phase as it can vary so much in length and regularity.

So, the short answer is that a study showed the average progression to be 1.9cm per hour[15]. The long answer is that it can last from anywhere from an hour or two to many days.

My own experience is that for my first labour it lasted three days. For my second it lasted about two hours!

You may ask: why is it so variable? There are many factors at play during labour and birth and the symphony of labour requires all of the instruments playing in concert together. If just one is out of sync it can throw the whole lot off course.

Factors that influence the progress (or not) of the latent phase include: levels of birth hormones in the mother, environmental factors, stress factors, position and movement of the mother, position of baby in pelvis (mal-position), position of baby's head (tilted up or down, or twisted), pelvis misalignment, fear in the mother, support available to mother, BMI of mother, other health factors, and the list goes on.[16]

First stage - established phase (active labour)

A woman is considered to be in established or active labour once she achieves a certain degree of dilation (around 4cm, although this can slightly vary in different hospitals) *in conjunction with* consistently regular contractions. This is usually the point at which you are advised to contact the hospital to arrange a midwife visit (home birth) or hospital assessment and admission.

This stage is measured by the pattern of contractions: if you have three complete contractions within 10 minutes consistently for 30–60 minutes then you would be assumed to have reached this phase although usually a vaginal examination would be used to verify this.

Generally, interruptions and changes of location (for example) don't tend to have a big impact on the pattern of labour – it is well established.

How can I tell I am in this phase?

Once you are having 90-second contractions every 2–3 minutes for half an hour or so, you are generally considered to be in active labour. As it is a combination of factors though, it is hard to be very specific and for some women they can display outward signs of being in established labour but not actually have progressed in terms of dilation at all, and for some it is the other way around!

Many midwives claim to be able to tell whether a woman is in established labour without even being in the room as often women get to a point where they need to fully focus on their contraction while it lasts, and make different kinds of sounds and noises in different stages.

Communication during a contraction becomes difficult or impossible as the intensity of the sensations requires all of your attention. You may be vocalising by this point as a way of coping with the contraction. You will often adopt a particular position or movement and a breathing pattern that show how fully absorbed you are in the contraction.

What is happening in the body?

The cervix is opening throughout this phase from around 4cm to full dilation – usually around 10cm, although this will depend on the size of the baby's head. The baby will also continue to rotate to face backwards in this phase.

The contractions will last up to 90 seconds and have maybe 2–3 minutes' rest in between. Women usually focus completely on the contraction and some may even keep their focus in between contractions.

How does it feel?

Contractions can feel like they are all-consuming in this phase. They can be intense, painful and require techniques to enable the mother to cope. By this point you have usually reached 'the zone' – when the primitive brain is in control and the rational brain has taken a back seat. Your consciousness can feel altered insofar as time seems to stretch and you can lose yourself somewhat in the experience of labour (and this is a great sign!).

What is tricky is that you can't really pinpoint with any accuracy whatsoever the shift from latent to established labour – it is very much a concept that we have introduced to allow us to gauge where we are in this stage.

This phase is often the point where some people might choose to take some pain relief, such as gas and air.

How long does it last?

Generally speaking, as far as the medical establishment is concerned, labour start time is calculated on the start of the established or active phase of labour, rather than the latent phase. This is because once labour is 'established', it is least likely to slow down or be significantly affected by outside factors.

Average active labours (and this includes the second stage so doesn't tell the whole story in terms of the first stage) are around 13 hours and dilation is around 1.3 cm per hour.[17]

That said, this is a generalisation and average statistic rather than a guideline. My own active labour was around 10 hours for my first baby and 90 minutes for my second!

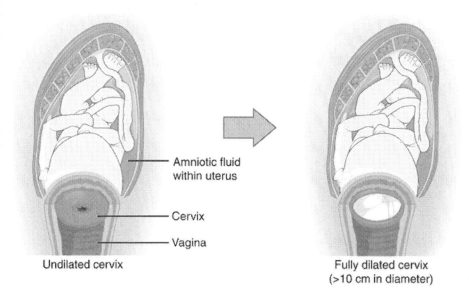

Amniotic fluid
within uterus

Cervix

Vagina

Undilated cervix

Fully dilated cervix
(>10 cm in diameter)

The cervix opening in the first stage of labour.

First stage: transition phase

As with the difference between latent and established labour in the first stage, the distinction between established labour and the start of transition can be blurred – although for some people it is very clear that they are in the transition phase.

How can I tell I am in this phase?

Sometimes contractions can slow down or stop completely during transition. Other times they can get longer and more intense. They can also stay the same! All of these are totally normal and just shows that the body is getting itself ready for birth.

Sometimes women find themselves letting out deep emotions during transition, and saying things that they may otherwise have filtered out. Due to the birth hormones rampaging through your body though, your inhibitions are lower and you might swear or be rude towards those close to you, or even express anxious thoughts.

What is happening in the body?

The end of the first stage marks the body's shift from opening the cervix, to preparing to expel the baby. During this phase, the baby will complete its rotation so that it is facing backwards. The cervix will also fully open by this phase, enough for the baby's head to pass through.

This phase is really marked by hormonal changes that are not directly physiological and so are shown more through behaviour than any outward signs.

How does it feel?

As mentioned above contractions can slow down or stop, get more intense or stay exactly the same.

If contractions stop then it is a great opportunity for rest and nourishment. If they get more intense then it is a really good sign that things are changing – hang in there!

The influence of adrenaline in the body can make you feel dizzy, sick, emotional, upset, anxious, or perhaps make you feel like you can't carry on.

It is common to hear women say such things as: [to father of baby] 'What have you done to me? I am never having sex with you ever again!', or 'I feel like I am going to die!', 'Make it stop', 'I just can't do this anymore!'

At this point the birth partner should be as supportive as possible and internally be saying to themselves: 'Wow, I think we may have hit transition. This is great news!'

How long does it last?

Transition is notoriously difficult to measure as the boundaries with established labour are so blurred. Coupled with the variable response (or not) of contractions and behaviour means that this stage is interpreted as much as measured.

We would consider anything up to 1–2 hours as normal, and beyond if all seems OK. Although, intervention may well be broached if it appears to last longer.

Second stage - foetal ejection reflex (pushing stage)

The onset of the second stage of labour, also known as the 'foetal ejection reflex',[18] is on the other hand, fairly easy to identify.[19] This stage is commonly referred to as the 'pushing stage' of labour but I really don't like this expression as it implies that the mother needs to actively push. We will see as we learn about birth physiology that this is not necessary as the uterus does all the pushing for you.

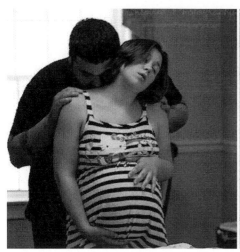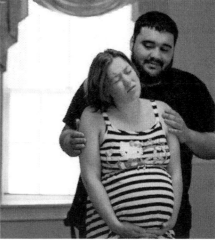

The support of the birth partner is key during transition.

How can I tell I am in this stage?

Usually the start of the second stage is accompanied by a clear and distinctive change in the sensations of contractions. It can literally feel like your body is pushing out the biggest, hardest poo you have ever had – without you being able to control it whatsoever!

What is happening?

The body has shifted the purpose of its contractions to quite literally ejecting the baby from the uterus. The uterus muscles push the baby out through the cervix, through the vagina, and then the head is born followed rapidly by the rest of the body.

How does it feel?

The quality of labour during the second stage can feel quite different than the first stage. Some women report second stage contractions as less painful, some more so than first stage. What is evident is that the body starts to spontaneously push out the baby and this feels different than before.

You can often really feel the baby's head coming down through the vagina, although it can sometimes seem that in between the contractions it goes back up – rest assured that every contraction helps the baby go further down through the vagina.

How long does it last?

This is widely variable from a few minutes to many hours! This could well be related to the mother's position and many other factors. After 2-3 hours, intervention would probably be discussed depending on concerns about the wellbeing of the mother and baby.

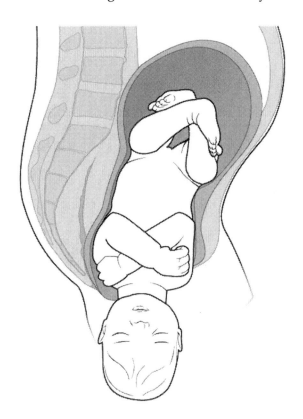

The baby is expelled from the body during the second stage.

Third stage - delivery of placenta

An often ignored stage of labour, the third stage is from the birth of the baby to the delivery of the placenta. Many people consider this to be a minor part of labour and interventions are routinely given here due to a lack of understanding about the importance of this stage. Midwives will watch a woman very closely during this stage as serious complications, while rare, can occur.

How can I tell I am in this stage?

It is easy to know if you are in this stage as your baby will have been born, but the placenta has not yet been delivered.

What is happening?

The contractions start again within about 10 minutes of the baby being born, albeit much shorter in duration and lower in intensity. The placenta detaches from the wall of the uterus and is delivered fairly easily.

How does it feel?

Many women claim not to even notice the contractions of the third stage as the reduction in intensity compared to the second stage is considerable. Couple this with the euphoria of cuddling your newborn baby and this is unsurprising!

You can feel the contractions, though, and in some cases, they can seem intense.

How long does it last?

On average the third stage of labour lasts anything between 5–60 minutes[20] in a mother left alone. It can last longer and this is often influenced by environmental and emotional factors that have an effect on the hormones involved.

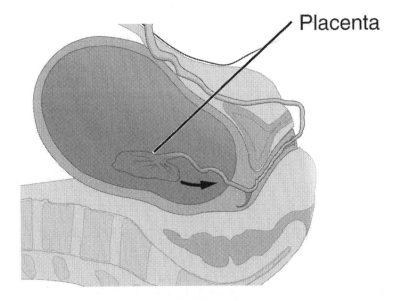

Placenta

The placenta is delivered once the baby is born.

Chapter 5
Planning Your Birth

Clearly there are many ways in which birth can need a bit of a helping hand – either though our own choices, or through medical necessity.

It can be incredibly overwhelming to remember everything and so creating birth preferences can be a great way to filter the information and tailor and personalise your preferences, both as a reference for yourself and also for your medical team.

It can be a really useful tool to help you research options for birth and decide what sounds good for you with regard to, for example, pain relief options, interventions, and optimal cord clamping.

There is a school of thought that planning birth is disingenuous and just sets the mother up for 'failure' if the birth doesn't go according to plan.

My personal opinion is that creating birth preferences helps to facilitate an environment in which to educate yourself about possibilities and choices in labour and birth. It gives both parents a sounding board to discuss options available to them.

It helps parents to get into the head space of labour and birth and start to visualise how it might be, and to get on the same page about what is important to them. If you can envisage scenarios and how you might react in them if that scenario happened, then you already have a strategy to deal with it.

But it is important to remember that it is not a shopping list. You can't plan labour or birth. Being open-minded about what might happen is the key to having a positive birth experience.

For many women, including myself, a traumatic birth can come as a direct result of reality not matching the 'fantasy'. Being fixated on having a certain sequence of events in your birth preferences that is what the 'perfect' birth looks like and not achieving it.

So, is there any point in having birth preferences? Yes, there is! It is helpful to be informed about what might happen during labour and after birth, and is helpful to highlight to yourself, your birth partner and your care providers what is really important to you.

Of course, the whole thing may go out of the window but any preparation for birth is useful in my opinion.

Read this book before creating your preferences

In some ways it doesn't make sense to put this chapter before you have informed and educated yourself about all the options covered in the plan.

In the overall context, though, it makes sense to include planning at the start!

My advice is to read the book first, then come back to this section to think about your birth preferences.

Birth Preferences Template

Before you start creating your birth preferences bear these points in mind.

1. You can't plan your birth. This is a summary of your birth *preferences* of the things you'd like to achieve or avoid, for example, optimal cord clamping.

2. Keep it simple. No more than one page of A4. (You could always create a longer version for you and your partner to refer to, but actually just covering key points should be enough).

3. Use bullets points, short sentences, and make it quick and easy to scan. There are many visual birth preferences out there, so have a look on the web if this suits your way of thinking.

4. Discuss it (in great detail) with your birth partner. Make sure you are on the same page (yes, pun intended!).

5. Be prepared to throw it out the window and go with the flow.

I have included a template below for you to use as a starting point. Feel free to copy and paste it and use it to write your own birth preferences but remember the golden rule: **You Can't Plan Your Birth**. This plan is also available in electronic format at www.birthzang.co.uk/2014/08/birth-preferences.

BIRTH PREFERENCES - YOUR NAME

Summary

Short summary sentence, e.g., 'My preferences outline my desire to experience an active labour and birth, remaining in an upright position. Of course, the main priority is delivering a healthy and happy baby and we will consider any action necessary to safeguard the baby's health.'

Bullet points of key preferences

- Include any relevant medical info, e.g., Blood type.
- Which pain relief you'd like to be offered or not.
- Birth pool?
- Delayed cord clamping.
- Natural 3rd stage.

Birth Companion/s

Name and relationship to you.

Birth Preparation

Describe any classes you've done or philosophy, e.g. Active Birth, Yoga, Hypnobirthing.

Pain relief

Your preferences about pain relief options, e.g.,

- I may wish to use gas and air.
- I do not wish to be offered Pethidine, or an epidural.

Labour and Birth

Summary of preferences for labour and birth:

- Minimal internal examinations.
- Birth position/not reclined.

- Birth pool.
- Episiotomy.
- Partner receive baby and tell me gender.

Care of Baby

- Optimal cord clamping until cord stops pulsing.
- Baby close by if needs resuscitation.
- Vitamin K – injection or oral.
- Immediate skin-to-skin.
- Breastfeeding.

Labour - 3rd Stage

- Natural 3rd stage.
- No Injection to deliver placenta ***again this needs to be highlighted and a good idea to tell your midwife as well. The injection is routinely given.***

Special Circumstances

If any special circumstances arise where you consider medical intervention necessary, please advise us of all options, including what should happen if we wait a little while longer, or do nothing (BRAIN).

Part 2
Medical Pain Relief

The most common forms of intervention in birth involve the use of medical pain relief options to help the mother cope with the sensations of labour and birth.

There are a huge number of non-medical options to help you cope including everything from holistic therapies such as acupuncture and reflexology, to adopting upright positions and avoiding lying on your back (see Active Birth techniques), to having a positive mindset.

While there are plenty of women who claim to have had pain-free births, some even experiencing orgasm during birth,[21] for many women the sensations of contractions can be extremely challenging.

When the statistics indicate that 44% of labours last less than 24 hours and 69.2% less than 48 hours,[22] it is clear that it can be a long and arduous process – it ain't called labour for nothing!

Experiencing the sensations of labour is a key part of the process. Pain helps us to understand physiology of labour, and also helps the body to regulate the process of labour by stimulating the production and secretion of the birth hormones. The two key birth hormones, oxytocin and endorphin, have a natural balancing act and if the first gets too strong, it inhibits the production of the second, thus ensuring that the body can always cope with the intensity of the contractions[23].

As with all sensations, there is an element of subjectivity; every woman will experience her labour differently. Certain factors predispose a woman to feel more intense sensations, such as posterior positioning of the baby (back-to-back), but as birth is such a complex recipe with different ingredients for each woman, you simply cannot predict how someone will cope.

If you have experienced a very long latent phase of labour – with many hours or days of contractions before achieving an established rhythm of labour – or went into labour after an exhausting day, late at night or while you are ill with a cold or flu (for example), you may well find that your tolerance to the sensations of labour is low.

The decision to opt for pain relief is a totally understandable one and if nearly 60% of births have some form of intervention (including anything except gas and air) then it is quite normal to choose a bit of help.

The decision to have pain relief should be based solely on the needs of the mother, rather than the perceived need by the birth partner or midwife. If you feel really strongly that you intend not to have any pain relief then you could state in your birth preferences that you do not want to be offered pain relief at all.

You could also agree a safe word or phrase with your birth partner to mean you *really* need pain relief. You have the right to change your mind at any time!

There are many ways to manage the pain and sensations of labour and birth.

I could (and probably will) write a book on all these different methods. Different things work for different people, as they experience labour sensations in different ways. Pain is not absolute – your environment and attitude can influence it and I heartily recommend doing research, attending antenatal classes and finding out all the ways you can enhance labour before considering medical pain relief.

But if there comes a time when it feels right to not let your pain cross over into suffering, then you can be confident knowing that you are making really informed choices.

Chapter 6
Tens Machine

Technically a TENS machine is not really a medical pain relief option, although many hospitals do have them to lend out and it is often the first thing that people reach for in labour. I felt it was relevant to include it here as while it could be considered natural insofar as it is not a drug, it nevertheless requires consideration before usage.

Some hospitals lend TENS machines but you can easily hire them or buy them from chemists and online for very reasonable costs. I would avoid buying a second-hand one to ensure that it works correctly.

I have also included some additional information in this chapter about whether or not a TENS machine actually works as there is some debate as to its efficacy, unlike stronger drug-based pain relief options.

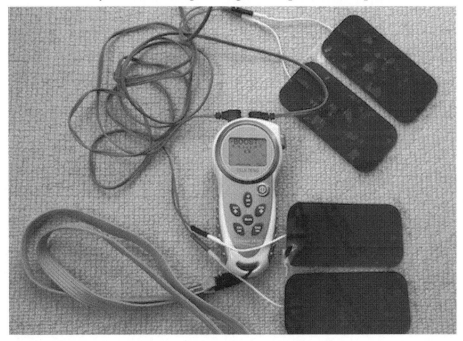

An Elle TENS machine, designed to be used in labour.

What is it?

TENS stands for Transcutaneous Electrical Nerve Stimulation.[24] It consists of a small battery-powered machine about the size of a mobile phone that produces a very small electrical current. You attach sticky pads to your skin and the electrical current is sent through your body from one set of pads to the other.

The electric current stimulates the nerves under the skin and it seems to work in two ways depending on the frequency of the current. A high current appears to confuse the nerve centres receiving pain signals and disrupt their transmission into the brain, thus 'reducing' the pain.

A low current is also thought to help stimulate the body's natural endorphins, again aiding the body in its own natural pain-relief system.

But does it actually work?

Well the crazy thing is that the answer to this is both a resounding *Yes* and a resounding *No*!

I did a (fairly unscientific) poll of mums on my Facebook network and out of 62 responses, discovered that

- 35% said it helped a bit
- 24% said it helped a lot
- 21% said it didn't help at all
- 18% said it was completely brilliant
- 2% said it was a complete waste of money!

So clearly there are a lot of differences of opinion about whether it works, although overall 75% of the mums polled reported positive results.

Looking at the comments these mums made, however, did shed some light on the situations where TENS machines were better or worse and enabled me to add some additional guidelines to use.

- Correct positioning of the pads made a big difference to its efficacy.
- It helps most when used early on in labour, so don't leave it too late to use it (this is probably because you need time to build up the endorphin levels).
- It was more of a distraction than pain relief.
- It really helped with a posterior labour (when your baby is back-to-back).

- It doesn't help very much for labours that come on fast and strong, or are induced (again the endorphins can't build up).
- You need to start at a low level and build it up slowly, rather than using a high frequency early on which is just annoying.

Here are a few comments that I feel sum up the consensus of opinion.

Briget: 'It was a distracting but not unpleasant feeling in the middle of a contraction, and that's what I needed.'

Marina: 'It did take the edge off from contractions but that was about it.'

Julie: 'It's only when I took it off did I realise how much it was helping in the early stages.'

What does science say?

This is where it gets very interesting. A 2009 Cochrane review of studies[25] looking at TENS machine use in labour concluded:

'There is only limited evidence that TENS reduces pain in labour and it does not seem to have any impact (either positive or negative) on other outcomes for mothers or babies. The use of TENS at home in early labour has not been evaluated. TENS is widely available in hospital settings and women should have the choice of using it in labour.'

So, there is no real evidence that it has any great effect, but that it is good to have as an option.

A further review in 2011,[26] reached the same conclusions and added:

'Although the guidelines of the National Institute for Health and Clinical Excellence recommend that TENS should not be offered to women in labour, women appear to be choosing it and midwives are supporting them in their choice. Given the absence of adverse effects and the limited evidence base, it seems unreasonable to deny women that choice. More robust studies of effectiveness are needed.'

No-one is telling women to use it and yet they are choosing to do so anyway and therefore more studies are needed.

Then I came across a damning article[27] from a well-respected organisation, Birth International, who claim that using a TENS machine in labour is nothing more than a 'marketing triumph' and is scathing even of the claims that a rise in endorphin level is occurring in labour:

'What about the claim that TENS increases endorphin levels and therefore is useful in encouraging natural birth? I have not seen any research that shows TENS increasing endorphin levels in labour. There may be some evidence

of increased endorphin levels when TENS is used in other situations (but I haven't found that either), but in any case, it would be unwise to assume from any such studies, that a similar effect would occur in labour, given that birth is a completely different physiological condition.'

Of course, just because there is no evidence does not always mean that is isn't working. Perhaps the studies have not actually looked at this particular aspect and have instead focussed on mums' pretty subjective reporting of their pain in labour (or their perception of it) often reflectively after the fact rather than at the time, so again adding even more to the subjectivity of the response.

Just a placebo effect?

So, then it looks as if using a TENS machine in labour has just a placebo effect. However, 75% of the mums I asked who had used a TENS machine said it helped them, even if only in a small way, so there must be something happening that is helping.

If it is just creating a distraction from the sensations of contractions, if it is just allowing a delay before using other pain relief options or interventions, if it is just giving you something to focus on during contractions, if it is just helping you feel in control of your labour… but if it works, who cares?

How do I use it?

As soon as labour starts you can start using the TENS machine. The gel pads come in pairs and you place each pair on your back, the top pair just around your bra line, either side of the spine, and the bottom pair around your knicker line just below the waistline on either side of the spine. The placement is quite important for effective use. You can reuse the gel pads a number of times (so you can take it off and put it back on again – ensure it is switched off first!) but it is advisable to have fresh pads if you have hired or borrowed the machine.

Each TENS machine is slightly different but they all have the same basic function. From the first contractions, you allow a continuous low current. This helps to boost the body's natural endorphins.

During a contraction, you increase the frequency and switch on the pain relief part of the TENS – stimulating the nerve signals to the brain and stopping the pain signals from getting through.

When the contraction has finished, you switch back to the low level current.

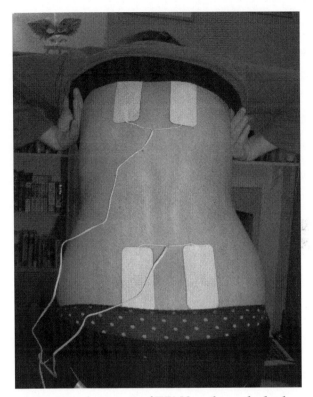

Showing the appropriate placement of TENS pads on the back.

You can set the intensity of the current at both the low and the high levels so you can build it up as labour builds in intensity.

TENS machines designed for labour also have a 'Boost' button so once you have set the higher level, when a contraction starts you can just hit the boost button and it will go to the higher level, making it very easy to use.

How does it feel?

Using a TENS machine feels a bit like someone is holding a couple of electric toothbrushes against your skin. It has a kind of buzzing feeling, a very fast and soft vibration. You feel it under the skin but it is not an unpleasant sensation.

The main area of sensation is the pads themselves. Some people find it really annoying, but many women have found it a really helpful tool in the earlier stages of labour.

When can't you use it?

It is not advised to use a TENS machine if you have a pacemaker or a heart rhythm disorder (such as arrhythmia or epilepsy), so please seek medical advice from your GP or consultant if this applies to you.

It is also not advisable to use a TENS machine on your abdomen during pregnancy, but it is fine to try it out on an arm or leg to figure out how it works before labour starts.

You should stick to the advised placing of the gel pads during labour, but you should never put the pads on your face or neck.

You can't use a TENS machine in water – it is an electrical device remember! – so if you have a shower or bath, or get into a birth pool you will need to remove it. Once you have finished and dried off, you can put it back on.

Some people find they are mildly allergic to the gel pads that stick to your back. The TENS has to have a moist connection to your skin so will only work if the gel is against your skin. You should also avoid putting the pads onto broken skin.

What are the Benefits?

The key benefits of a TENS machine are that:

- It is fully controlled by the mother.
- There are no side effects (unless medically contraindicated)
- It can be stopped at any time.
- It can be mobile.
- It can be used in conjunction with other pain relief.
- It can be hired/bought by mother, and used at home from the onset of labour with no prescription required.
- It can be used at home, in a midwife-led birthing centre or hospital.

What are the Risks?

The amazing thing about a TENS machine is that it has absolutely minimal side effects! This means it is completely safe for you and completely safe for your baby.

Of course, there are a few risks, although they appear to be far outweighed by the benefits.

- There are some medical conditions that are contraindicated. Seek medical advice if you have a pacemaker or a heart rhythm disorder (such as arrhythmia or epilepsy).
- It only offers mild pain relief.
- It can cause skin irritation if you have sensitive skin.
- It doesn't always provide the right type of or enough relief.

Are there any Alternatives?

There aren't really any direct alternatives to a TENS machine, other than hands-on massage.

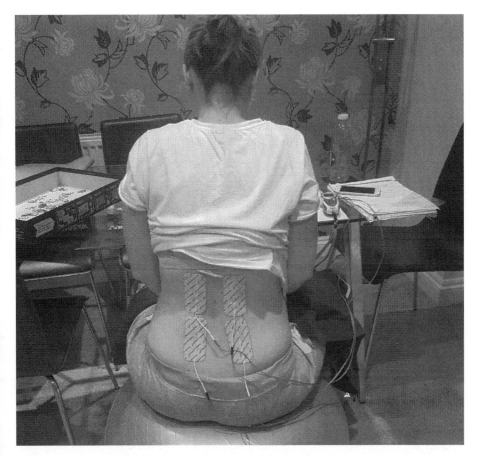

Siobhan found the TENS machine useful in early labour and used it while distracting herself with a large jigsaw!

What are the Implications?

The great thing about a TENS machine is it has no lasting effects and therefore does not lead to further interventions.

The key issues are that it can't be used in water, so if you are planning to have a bath, shower or use a birth pool, then you need to remove it. As water provides a degree of pain relief anyway, the benefits of getting in water would probably outweigh removing the TENS machine, and you can always get out of the water and put it back on if you change your mind.

Faulty machines can also cause electric shocks so make sure you hire or buy one from a reputable source.

What if I do Nothing?

You can certainly do without a TENS machine and as people tend not to have many labours it is very hard to know if it helps compared to if you didn't use one.

With most benign pain relief options, the choice is up to you if you use it and how you feel you are coping/can cope.

How can I minimise complications?

- Make sure you are not exposed to water.
- Use the TENS early in labour and don't take it off.
- Practice using it before labour starts (on your arm or leg).

REAL EXPERIENCE: *Laura's Story*

I used a TENS machine from the time that the contractions started and found it really helpful – especially as I kept finding different settings to adjust as the contractions got stronger! (We hadn't gotten around to reading the instructions properly before I went into labour.)

I also used gas and air at the hospital and was glad I'd been told beforehand that it makes you feel light-headed/ slightly drunk. It didn't make me feel sick though as it does for some people.

For the actual birth, I was in a birth pool. I was nervous about having to stop using the TENS but the water at that stage was just as effective at reducing pain.

REAL EXPERIENCE: *Lucrezia's Story*

With my second labour, I had contractions all day and as soon as I realised, I popped my TENS machine on. Instant relief.

When my contractions got stronger I upped the strength of the machine. It got me through the whole day and managed to have a relatively normal day with my toddler.

In the evening the contractions got more regular and I went straight to hospital. It turns out I was too far gone and the only pain relief I could have was the good old gas and air. That got me through my very short and intense labour and through my stitching downstairs afterwards too. I would definitely recommend it.

Chapter 7
Gas and Air (Nitrous Oxide)

What is it?

This is a gas that is comprised of 50% nitrous oxide and 50% oxygen that is inhaled during contractions to relieve pain. The most common brand name for this is Entonox[28], but it is commonly known as 'gas and air'.[29] Nitrous oxide is also known as laughing gas, but mixing it with oxygen makes it less powerful, safer and concentrates the side effects to pain relief rather than laughing.

It is also used for other medical procedures where short-term pain relief is required, such as suturing perineal damage after birth, and other non-birth-related situations.

It is stored in metal cylinders and administered via tubes to a nozzle placed in the mouth.

How do I use it?

You breathe through a demand valve via a plastic nozzle to inhale the gas and exhale air. The demand valve is similar in concept to one used during Scuba diving so you keep the nozzle in your mouth while both inhaling and exhaling. When you inhale, you take in the gas. As you exhale the valve releases the breath to the room.

It takes about 30 seconds to take effect and wears off within 60 seconds of stopping inhaling it. It works best when you inhale as soon as you feel the contraction is starting so its maximum efficacy is coordinated with the most painful part of the contraction. You can either stop inhaling in between contractions or use it continuously.[30]

Its use may be restricted in the second stage of labour to help the mother focus on birth.

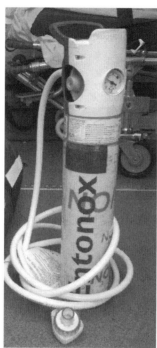

A cylinder of Entonox with a demand valve nozzle (bottom of image).

How does it feel?

After 15–30 seconds of inhalation, you start to feel the effects of gas and air. It acts to dull the sensations of labour, but doesn't take them away completely. Many people describe it more as taking the edge off the pain to make it manageable.

People experience it in different ways – some positive, some not so much – but it can make you feel a bit giddy and slightly high, but never out of control.

Excessive use of gas and air, or usage after a long latent labour when the mother is tired and hungry can result in more negative side effects.

When can you use it?

It is a mobile resource and midwives who attend home births will usually have a cylinder for use in their kit.

It is generally best avoided in the very early stages of labour and used when the mother feels that she has used all her natural methods of pain relief and resources, and once her labour is fully established.

If you are having a hospital birth then you wouldn't be admitted until you were in established labour and so you wouldn't have access until then anyway.

When can't you use it?

Nitrous oxide should not be used if you have a bowel obstruction, pneumothorax, middle ear and sinus disease, and following cerebral air-contrast studies.[31]

What are the Benefits?

As the first port of call for most people when it comes to medical pain relief, gas and air has many benefits.

- It acts really quickly, taking effect within seconds.
- It helps to take the edge off strong contractions.
- It can be stopped at any time with no lasting effects – within 60 seconds the effects have gone completely.
- It can be used for the duration of labour, and afterwards if required.
- It does cross the placenta but has no known side effects on the baby.
- You are not required to have monitoring with it.
- It is really versatile – it can be used at home, in a birth pool, in any position.
- It is controlled by the mother and is easy to use.
- It helps the mother to regulate her breathing and get into a good rhythm which is helpful for natural pain relief.
- It can be used at a home birth, in a midwife-led birthing centre or hospital.

What are the Risks?

- Clamping the teeth onto the mouthpiece can cause a stiff jaw and this could also have an effect on the cervix.[32]
- If it is used continuously for many hours, you can get a bit 'high'.
- It can cause dry mouth and lips – you can mitigate this by sipping water and using lip salve.

- It can cause nausea and sickness in some cases.

- It can also make you laugh or tearful.

- It is only a mild painkiller and so further pain relief may be required.

- Inhaling nitrous oxide for longer than a 24-hour period may affect white cell production and vitamin B12 action. An assessment, as well as a discussion with the woman, is needed to determine the duration of use.

- Entonox does cross the placenta, but is rapidly eliminated when the woman ceases inhalation. It does not affect the foetus.[33]

- Used in conjunction with diamorphine or pethidine, it could increase the likelihood of negative side effects.

Are there any Alternatives?

In terms of short-term pain relief that is easily administered and controlled by the mother, and has a very short duration of effect, there are no other pain relief options in this category, other than the TENS machine.

There are indeed many natural ways of dealing with the sensations of labour and you could certainly try as many of these as possible before choosing gas and air.

What are the Implications?

Once you have started gas and air, you probably won't stop (or want to stop) so it is best to wait until you feel you really need it until picking up the nozzle.

It just takes the edge off the sensations of contraction so if you use it too early in labour, or if your labour is prolonged, then you may feel that you require additional pain relief later on.

There are no other real implications; its use does not lead to any further complications and is very popular for that reason.

What if I do Nothing?

Taking gas and air is very much a choice and many women are perfectly capable of coping with labour with no pain relief at all.

It really depends on how well you feel you are coping with the sensations of labour.

By delaying the use of gas and air you may well find new and different ways of coping with labour and finding reserves of energy. The great thing is that you can use it at any point where you feel you need it and stop at any time if you don't like it.

How can I minimise complications?

- Keep your jaw soft – don't clamp and tense the jaw.
- Keep well hydrated with sips of water (but remember to go to the toilet!).
- Keep lips soft with lip balm.
- Only use it for contractions.
- Start to breathe in as soon as a contraction is coming.

REAL EXPERIENCE: Anna's Story

Both my labours were pretty fast. Active labour was less than four hours. I used gas and air for both, although I was very, very reluctant for my first and managed nearly three hours without anything.

Mainly I was worried it would make me sick and I have a phobia of vomit. It didn't. Got right on it with my second baby. It was a massive relief and helped immensely.

Then my midwife took away the gas and air when I was fully dilated and I had to use the contraction 'pain' to push otherwise I think I would have just happily kept using the gas and air to get me through for a lot longer.

I pushed for 11 minutes for my first baby and 8 minutes, my second – because the contraction pain was so intense. The gas and air really had dulled the contractions really well for me.

I couldn't and wouldn't keep still. I had to keep moving.

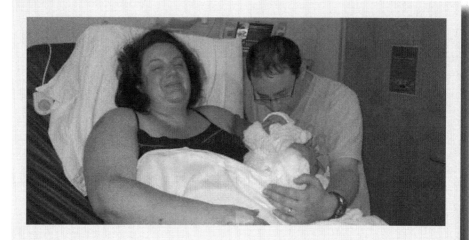

First baby I was on all fours then up-right on the bed – I just couldn't be on my back. They wanted to give me an epidural, but when they checked I was too far gone and Poppy would be born before they could do it.

My fluids were monitored through the cannula as well as medication for pre-eclampsia.

The placenta was out about 10 minutes after and I remember thinking it felt like having a poo. No stitches or tearing. I then had postpartum haemorrhaging after Poppy was born. I used the gas and air because they had to remove the blood clots in my womb by pushing on my tummy.

This was worse than the labour and birth and I passed out. I lost nearly 4 pints, but didn't need a blood transfusion.

Second baby I had attended pregnancy yoga and again I couldn't keep still. I did a lot of squatting and rocking. I had my baby in a squat position on the bed. I think the moving about helped my labour.

If I had to keep still I am 100% certain I would have had other pain relief/intervention.

Chapter 8
Intradermal Water Blocks
(Sterile Water Injections)

What is it?

These are injections of sterile water[34] just under the skin in the back to help relive back pain in labour (usually as a result of a posterior/back-to-back baby). It is thought to slow down or block the signals from the back and uterus up to the brain through nerves in the skin, although it is not very well understood.[35]

How do I use it?

Minute amounts of sterile water are injected just under the skin in the back, from 0.1–0.5ml per injection. Four injections are made into the sacral/lumbar region of the back, although the exact site seems not to be that important. [36] The injections can be repeated as required.

How does it feel?

The initial injection feels like a wasp sting and can be painful, which is why they try to administer two injections simultaneously by two members of staff.

This initial sting rapidly ceases and women report to have relief from back pain fairly quickly, lasting up to 120 minutes.[37]

When can you use it?

It is generally used in established labour when labour sensations are experienced intensively in the back. If your baby is lying in a posterior position, the labour pain often presents across the lower back. It is administered when pain is considered unbearable, possibly as an alternative to an epidural.

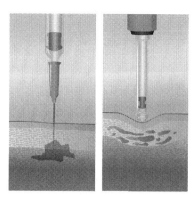

Intradermal injection

When can't you use it?

If you don't have back pain in labour, then this wouldn't be offered. It probably wouldn't be administered if you had any skin issues or sores, although there aren't any clear guidelines as to contraindications.

What are the Benefits?

The injections are quick to administer and are fast-acting – some women reported relief in the next contraction.

- They can be administered by a midwife so can be done very soon after being requested.
- They can be used at any time in labour.
- There appear to be no known side effects for the mother or baby as it is an injection of water rather than a drug.
- You can have multiple doses as required.
- It does not affect your mobility, how you feel your labour sensations and ability to push, or need for other pain relief.
- No additional monitoring is required.
- It can be used in a midwife-led birthing centre, or hospital.

What are the Risks?

Administering the injections is quite painful and can cause swelling, soreness or slight bleeding on the site of the injection, or even an infection if the site is not kept clean.[38]

Once the injection is administered you can't stop it – you have to wait for it to wear off naturally (up to 120 minutes).

It may not work or wear off very quickly.

There is no clear evidence that this treatment actually works, other than the anecdotal evidence from women undertaking the injections.[39] But, as with the TENS machine, a placebo effect can still be a powerful pain reliever.

Are there any Alternatives?

Similar alternatives don't really exist. Some believe that the injections are analogous to acupuncture which could be considered an option, although as the site of the injections doesn't seem to be relevant this probably means that acupuncture is not comparable.

A TENS machine is probably the closest alternative.

You could also consider trying to shift the baby's position out of a posterior one by using movement, yoga postures or rebozo (a type of large scarf used in labour) to encourage the baby to rotate into a better position that may alter the focus of sensations.

What are the Implications?

There are no obvious implications for this treatment as while it is not technically a medical pain relief option as it is not a drug administered, it is only offered in the hospital setting.

It has no effect on other pain relief options.

What if I do Nothing?

The pain in the back will continue and may intensify. You may need to find alternative ways to cope with these sensations, or find a way to help the baby move.

How can I minimise complications?

- Ask for injections to be administered by two staff.
- Ensure the site of the injection is kept clean.

REAL EXPERIENCE: *Katie's Story*

My waters started to break when I went to bed at 11pm but I didn't really have any pain until an hour or so later, and used the TENS quite early on – ramping it up as it went along.

I had a brief early visit to the hospital just to set my mind at rest that all was well and was told then that the baby was back-to-back. For me, the TENS was really helpful and together with a strong back massage from my husband meant I could stay at home until the contractions were very close together. It just seemed to interfere with my back pain which became very intense.

When I reached the hospital at 9am, I was relieved to be 8cm dilated but was finding the pain less manageable so the midwife gave me four water injections in my back.

They were a lot more painful to have than I expected. Whether the effects are like a placebo I'm really not sure but I was happy to try something different at that stage, and it did seem to help. I suppose that being able to choose to do something positive that might help gave me a mental boost when I really needed it. And the fact that it is drug free very much appealed to me.

I also had gas and air but not sure I was using it properly during labour – I guess it was helpful to calm my breathing but I could probably have found a better way of doing that.

I did have gas and air for my stitches afterwards and used it a lot more and whilst mildly effective, did make me feel quite drunk and sick though this didn't last long.

Overall, I was very happy that I was able to have the natural pool birth I had hoped for, and the support of the midwife was great. I suppose my biggest surprise was how quickly time went. I was in the pool for about an hour and a half before Joshua was born at 11am but it honestly felt like 20 mins... I have no idea where that time went.

Chapter 9
Opioid-based Pain Relief

What is it?

There are various options for opioid-based pharmacological relief from labour pain. Diamorphine, Pethidine and Meptazimole are the most commonly encountered ones. They are all morphine-based drugs administered for pain relief in labour by changing the nerve receptors in your brain.

The drug doesn't take away the pain but affects your consciousness and how you experience the pain – it sedates you.

Diamorphine is basically heroin, an opiate made from morphine derived from the Poppy.[40]

Pethidine is a synthetic opioid that was developed in 1939 for medical use.[41] It is the cheapest out of all of the opioids mentioned, and also one of the strongest.

Meptazimole (or Meptid) is a more recently developed opioid analgesic developed in the 1970s. It tends to have a shorter onset but also wears off more quickly.

Hospitals usually have one that they prefer to administer and so you will usually just be offered their standard one.

I am going to base this section on the use of pethidine as it is most commonly used, and cover the others in the 'Alternatives' section below. The benefits and risks are quite similar and I will outline the differences in this section.

You can find out which drug your hospital offers by asking your midwife or maternity unit.

How do I use it?

A midwife will inject the drug into your leg muscle. It usually takes around 20 minutes to start working and the effects last between 2–4 hours.

It can be repeated once more if necessary later in the labour.

How does it feel?

Pethidine is a sedative and can make you feel quite drowsy, but allows you to rest and relax, helping time to pass more quickly. It does not take away the pain of labour, but works on your endorphin receptors in the brain, changing the way you experience it.

There are quite a lot of doubts as to how effective it is as a pain relief option, with some women reporting that it made no difference to the pain but made them feel they were out of control.[42] Some women find it gives them just enough relief to get them through a few more hours, or to get some rest.

When can I use it?

You can use it once you are in labour, although most midwives would wait until you were in established labour to administer it. If you are still in an early stage of labour, once it wears off you may be able to have a subsequent dose.

When can't I use it?

Pethidine is not given once your cervix is fully dilated (10cm) or if the baby is expected to be born in the next hour. This is because it has a strong effect upon the baby at birth and so the aim is for all the effects to have worn off by the time the baby is born.

What are the Benefits?

Pethidine offers a strong dose of pain relief, much stronger than the other forms of pain relief already discussed in previous chapters.

- It can be given in early labour when an epidural would not be administered.
- The dose can be adjusted to suit the mother's needs.
- Subsequent doses can be administered.
- Pethidine won't slow down your labour.

- It can help you postpone an epidural.[43]
- You don't need additional monitoring.

What are the Risks?

Pethidine is a really strong drug and there are many risks associated with it.

- It has to be administered in the delivery suite.
- You can't get into water for 2 hours afterwards.[44]
- There is only a small window of time when this drug is effective and can be used.
- You can appear outwardly normal but feel out of control.
- Common side effects are: dizziness, drowsiness, nausea or sickness.[45]
- It can make you feel drowsy and want to lie down which makes other interventions more likely as lying down does not encourage labour to progress.
- Some women report that it doesn't take away the pain but makes you feel 'out of your head' or even hallucinate.
- If you don't like the effects of the drug you have to just wait and bear it until it wears off.
- More serious/unusual side effects are: respiratory depression, hypotension, hypothermia, tremors, hallucinations, confusion, anxiety, nervousness and vertigo. It goes without saying that none of these side effects will enhance your labour!
- The key difference in risks to other options already discussed is that Pethidine and opiates do have a big effect on the baby.[46]
- It affects alertness of baby and can affect their Apgar score (this measures the baby's condition at birth and helps assess if further special care is required).
- It can affect independent breathing in the baby.
- It takes many hours to work its way out of the mother's system – it could still affect the baby even after it has worn off in the mother.
- It could impact breastfeeding and bonding with the baby.

This is not even a comprehensive list of all the side effects and known complications (just the most common ones) and it is advisable to do further research on these drugs before making a decision to use them, particularly if you have a medical condition that could be a contraindication.

Are there any Alternatives?

The other opioids that you may encounter are:

- Diamorphine: said to be a more effective painkiller than pethidine, but can affect the baby's breathing.
- Meptazinole (Meptid): less likely to affect the baby, but can cause more nausea and vomiting in the mother.
- Morphine Sulphate (Oramorph): offered to women experiencing very painful contractions in early labour. It helps them rest and conserve energy and can even go home until their labour progresses.
- Remifentaril: used if the mother is contraindicated for an epidural.

What are the Implications?

You would usually need a vaginal examination before having Pethidine to have a clear idea of the cervical progression of labour.

If you are feeling drowsy and unwell, then it may affect your ability to maintain upright positions and follow your body's instincts in movements and natural ways to cope with labour. This drowsiness can also affect your ability to make further decisions and choices about your labour.

If the Pethidine wears off and pain is still severe but you are too late to have an epidural, then you may find your experience of labour is much worse once the drugs wear off.

What if I do Nothing?

Most people choose opioid pain relief as they feel they are not coping well with the sensations of labour and want to avoid an epidural if they can.

Avoiding this pain relief takes away the risks, but also means you need to find other ways to cope with the sensations of labour.

How can I minimise complications?

- Ask for a low dose to see if it is right for you.
- If you experience side effects and need to lie down, try to stay lying on your side to maintain pelvic mobility, and prop up your upper body to maintain gravity.

REAL EXPERIENCE: Siobhan's Story

My labour lasted 4 days from Friday morning to Monday lunch time. I wasn't admitted until the Sunday evening so during my time at home I used the TENS Machine and took several baths. Whilst the TENS Machine didn't take the pain away it was a good distraction... I managed to complete a 1000-piece jigsaw puzzle using the machine!

By the time we were admitted, I was exhausted but only 3cm so was given a shot of diamorphine to help me get some rest. Diamorphine wasn't what I expected, it didn't take away the pain but I felt pretty woozy and drunk which allowed me to doze between contractions.

Finally, on the Monday morning active labour kicked off and we went to delivery. I had asked for a drug called Remifentanil at this stage as I was unable to have an epidural because of a gestational blood disorder, however my wonderful midwife talked me out of having it and encouraged me to manage with just gas and air as she thought it would be only a few hours before Joshua was born (she was right).

Given how the diamorphine made me feel I'm glad I didn't end up taking another opioid. Once I got used to using the gas and air that was enough to get through each contraction.

Once I started pushing, my midwife made the decision to give me an episiotomy as she expected me to tear and she was right again. I ended up with a 3rd degree tear, if she hadn't performed the episiotomy I dread to think how bad the tear would have been. At 12:16pm Joshua was born, wide eyed and ready to experience the world.

It's great to have an idea of what you want and do not want in labour for pain relief but be open-minded about changing your choices once you're in labour, remembering always that the end goal is a healthy baby and a healthy mum.

I wish I had the opportunity to read real-life testimonials about certain types of pain relief and how it did/didn't work. Whilst no two experiences are the same, I would have felt a little more prepared for the way my body reacted to pain relief.

Chapter 10
Epidural or Spinal Block

What is it?

This is an injection of a local anaesthetic drug around your lumbar spine region. The anaesthetic is injected into the space in between the vertebra of your spine and spinal fluid (known as the epidural area) in order to numb the nerves in the lower half of the body and reduce or remove pain from the area.[47] In fact, 'epidural' refers to the place in the body in which the drugs are administered rather than the drug itself.[48]

The drugs used in an epidural come under the category of local anaesthetics such as Bupivacaine, Chloroprocaine, or Lidocaine, and can be combined with some narcotics, such as Epinephrine, Fentanyl, Morphine, or Clonidine to enhance the anaesthetic affect. The specific drugs and combination of drugs will vary across hospitals so it is best to check with your midwife or maternity unit as to the exact combination they use.[49]

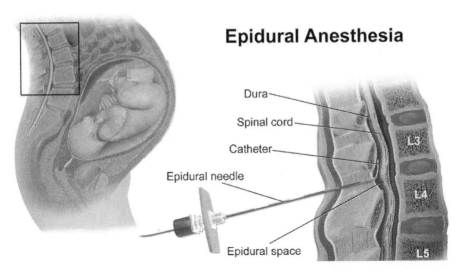

Epidural Anesthesia

Dura

Spinal cord

Catheter

Epidural needle

Epidural space

L3

L4

L5

An epidural administered in the lumbar region of the back into the epidural space.

The difference between a spinal block and an epidural is that the spinal block is one injection to administer a single dose of the drug(s), and an epidural is an injection to place a very thin catheter into the epidural space and remains in place so the drug can be administered continuously for as long as required.

There is also a mobile or walking epidural used in some hospitals that uses a lower dose of the drug and is self-administered via a catheter. It enables you to retain some sensation and movement and raise or lower the dosage to suit your requirements, although actually walking is probably not possible, especially if you use it for a prolonged period of time as the drugs build up in your system.[50] This type of epidural is not that common in the UK and your hospital would be able to advise you if this was on offer.

How do I use it?

You are usually asked to stop using gas and air while the injections are being administered.

Firstly, a cannula is inserted in the back of your hand or wrist to administer IV fluids and drugs to avoid low blood pressure.

You have to sit up over the side of a bed and bend forwards over your belly while hunching your shoulders or lie on your side. You need to keep very still, which can be challenging when you are having intensive contractions.

Your back is cleaned and for a spinal block an injection is administered in the spinal cord area.

Alternatively, for an epidural, a thin needle is inserted into your back. This needle is immediately removed and leaves behind a fine plastic tube (catheter) into your back to continually administer the anaesthetic. The tube is then taped into place.

The drugs take about 15–20 minutes to start working. The spinal block and mobile epidural last for around 1–2 hours before starting to wear off. The epidural will last for as long as the drug is administered and will take some hours to wear off after the drugs are stopped.

If you have a mobile epidural, there will be a button to press to administer a further dose when you feel you need to top it up.

You will also have a catheter inserted into your urethra as your bladder muscles are numbed. This ensures you can wee.

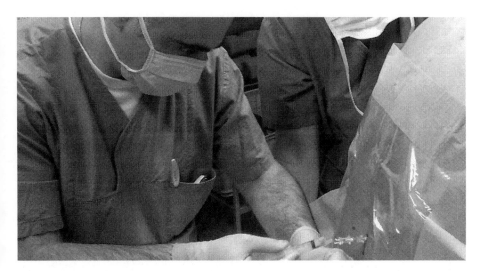

An epidural is administered by an anaesthetist.

How does it feel?

The administration of the drugs via injection are quite uncomfortable and sitting still while having the injections is also challenging as it can mean you have to stay still for 5–15 minutes.

Once the drugs kick in you will not be able to move properly or feel pain from around the waist down. If you have had a spinal block for a forceps delivery or caesarean, this numbness may start higher up the body and include the chest and breast area.

You may feel pressure in the area but no pain, a bit like when you have your mouth numbed at the dentist.

With a mobile epidural, you may still have some sensation and move-ment in the legs as the nerves are not numbed so much. To begin with you may well be able to walk, however the more doses you have and the longer you have the mobile epidural, the more the numbness builds up and you become less and less mobile, and perhaps a bit groggy due to the higher levels of narcotics.[51]

When can I use it?

You can have an epidural once you are in established labour, around 4–5cm dilated. It can be administered earlier if the labour is very pro-longed and the mother is getting exhausted.

It is usually the last resort for most mothers when they just feel that they can't cope any more with the sensations of labour, or are so exhausted that they need to rest.

In the case of a spinal block or mobile epidural, you could let the drugs wear off to be more involved in the second (pushing) stage of labour.

A spinal block would be used if there was a known period of time that anaesthesia was required, for example a caesarean section, an assisted delivery, or if you are quite well dilated.

An epidural would be used if the period of time required is likely to be longer than an hour or two.

When can't I use it?

An epidural is unlikely to be given if you were nearly or at 10cm dilated or in the second stage of labour. This is due to the fact it takes time to arrange for it to be administered, and also for the drug effects to kick in.

There are also certain medical conditions that are contraindicated for using an epidural.[52] This will obviously vary depending on the type and combination of drugs involved.

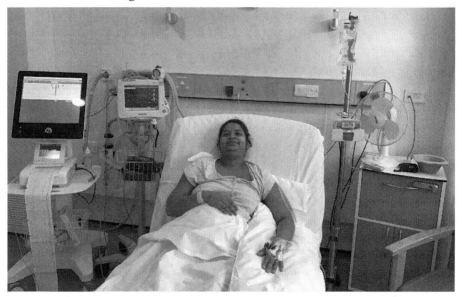

Jyoti found great relief after having an epidural.

Contraindications include:

- Active maternal haemorrhage.
- Septicaemia or fever.

- Thrombocytopenia, or low platelets (although this is dependent on the platelet count level).

- Infection on or near the site that the injection will be administered.

- Neurologic disease or condition, such as multiple sclerosis or spina bifida.

- Coagulopathy.[53]

- Allergy to local anaesthetics.

- Taking medicines to thin your blood, such as warfarin.[54]

- Blood-clotting abnormality that increases your risk of bleeding.

- Previous back surgery, or other problems with your back.

- Spinal deformity or severe arthritis in your spine.

What are the Benefits?

Epidurals provide full pain relief for 85% women and the pain is completely removed. There are no effects to your consciousness – no drowsiness or feeling of disorientation – and the pain is significantly lessened or removed – you basically feel back to normal.

This means that you are able to rest, sleep, eat and recuperate. It also brings you out of the deep focussed zone of labour and so decision-making is easier.

It can be reduced for the second stage, so that you can have a rest and then continue and finish your labour more naturally.

Some studies have shown that use of an epidural can lower the risk of postnatal depression.[55]

There have also been indications that the mother breathes better with an epidural and that lower levels of stress hormones are released which can cause distress in the baby.

Most women report a great sense at relief when the epidural starts to take effect.[56]

In one study, it showed that only 1% women needed additional pain relief after the epidural was successfully administered, in comparison with 28% who used other pain relief options.[57]

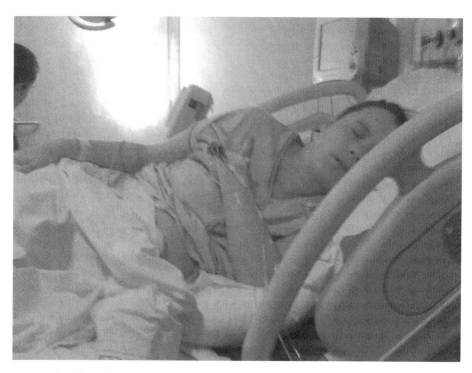

An epidural can help you get some much-needed rest.

What are the Risks?

An epidural or spinal block is administered by an anaesthetist and so there may be some delay between requesting one and it being administered depending on the availability of the anaesthetist.

There is also a chance that the injection does not place the drugs in quite the right place, the anaesthetic does not distribute evenly or the catheter falls out, and so the effects wear off very quickly, or don't kick in and it needs to be repeated (up to 15%).[58]

With a mobile epidural, the drugs used have a combination using more narcotic and less anaesthetic, so while there is less numbness but more pain relief, it can leave you feeling drowsier as a result, especially after multiple doses.

There are a number of common side effects to an epidural, some more common than others. Some of these side effects can last for months after the epidural itself.

- Drop in blood pressure (14%), this can lead to

  o Dizziness and nausea.

- Fever (23%).
- Numbness or tingling in legs (nerve stimulation/damage).
- Difficulty or problems urinating (15%).
- Punctures the dura (protective layer around spinal cord), causing fluid to leak. This can cause headaches lasting anything up to a few days (1%)
- Back pain at the site of injection.
- Skin pain at site of injection.
- Infection at site of injection.
- Itchy skin.

An epidural does hold some extremely rare, but quite serious compilations. The NHS website indicates, 'The best estimate of the overall risk of permanent harm from an epidural in labour is between 1 in 80,000 and 1 in 320,000.'

- Epidural haematoma – a collection of blood in the epidural space as a result of broken blood vessels. This is very rare but can result in very serious complications including paraplegia.
- Nerve damage 1/1000 can last more than 6 months.
- Infection or clot 1/50,000.
- Seizure.
- Cardiac arrest or death.

Because an epidural is an opioid, it has an effect on the hormonal processes of labour and birth. This is discussed more in the section below on the implications of epidural, but it can slow labour down and increase the risk of further interventions.

These are a summary of the risks but obviously, they will vary depending on the exact cocktail of drugs used with the epidural. It is highly advisable to seek more information from your hospital and fully research the particular drugs involved.

Epidurals also have an effect on the baby and the drugs go through to baby's bloodstream, although there do not appear to be any long-term disadvantages to the baby.

- It can make it harder for baby to get in correct position for birth (due to lying on your back).
- The baby may have a slower heart rate.

- The baby may find it hard to regulate their temperature once born.

Are there any Alternatives?

An epidural is really the last line of pain relief for labour and birth and there are few alternatives.

If you have low blood platelets or other contraindications for epidural, then you may be offered an alternative drug called Remifentanil. This is more analogous to an opioid drug than an epidural in its effects, although it is administered via intravenous drip and is controlled by the mother as the effects wear off within 3–5 minutes.[59]

The mobile epidural does allow you to move more (potentially) although is not always available.

The spinal block – just one injection that wears off – rather than continuous intravenous delivery would potentially have fewer side effects due to the administration not involving a catheter, although the actual effects of the drugs are similar.

In truth, there are not any real alternatives to epidurals, and while the risks can seem large and many, the benefits in terms of pain relief are also significant.

What are the Implications?

There are numerous implications of the epidural, some implications are guaranteed and some of them just give an increased risk of a further possibility of intervention. There are plenty of studies that do not show a link with increased rates of caesarean or effect on the newborn, although anecdotal evidence and information provided by services (such as the NHS) imply that there could be implications that just haven't been properly documented.

Implications that are guaranteed are as follows.

- An epidural is not administered at a home birth or midwife-led unit, and so you would need to transfer to a hospital delivery suite.

- You and your baby will need continuous monitoring. With a mobile epidural, this could further affect the mother's mobility.

- Mother requires a catheter into the bladder as bladder function is lost. The catheter remains until after the birth (12 hours after the last top-up) and the mother will be required to provide a sizeable urine sample before she is discharged from hospital to ensure there is no damage to the urethra.

- Mother requires a cannula in the hand/wrist to administer IV fluids.

- Movement is restricted (mobile epidural) or impossible. The drugs numb the nerves from the waist down (or chest), so the sensation is lost in the lower half of the body and it is effectively paralyzed.

- The standard epidural takes 2–4 hours to wear off after the drugs have stopped being administered – admission to a postnatal ward in hospital after birth would be necessary until the drugs have worn off, and the mother has been given a clean bill of health. (In a birth with no complications, the mother can be discharged as soon as she and her baby have been checked by a Doctor, although many women opt to be admitted to a postnatal ward for a day or so.)

- An epidural makes labour last longer – while studies show that the overall length of labour is only slightly affected (and anyway, how can you truly measure how long a labour might have been had an intervention not taken place?), it is clear that epidural drugs have an effect on the hormones and physiology of birth.

Possible implications:

- You may need to have the epidural administered more than once to take full effect, if it doesn't work the first time or has been incorrectly administered.

- The hormones of birth (oxytocin, prolactin) can be suppressed. This could have a number of effects including: slowing the labour down, making contractions weaker which would have an effect on the rate the cervix dilates and the body's ability to expel the baby in the second stage. The mother's endorphin levels at birth are also lowered, which could affect bonding and overall satisfaction of the birth. Establishing breastfeeding successfully could also be affected as it is primarily a hormonal process.[60]

- The mother usually has to adopt a supine/reclined position and this has an effect on the utilisation of gravity in birth. Gravity can assist in the correct positioning of baby and also aiding the baby's descent through the pelvis in the second stage.

- The pelvic floor muscles are immobilised. They assist the baby to get into the correct position for birth and assist in the expulsion of the baby in the second stage.

- The pelvis is immobilized and when in a reclined supine position, the pelvis is held in a closed position, reducing the space for the baby to pass through. This could create a longer second stage and possible complications, such as shoulder dystocia, although studies show differing results.

- The mother can't feel the urge to push – makes it very hard to push baby out as you have no feedback from your body.

- There have been a number of studies that show a greater chance of assisted delivery (forceps or ventouse) with an epidural, no doubt due to the effect on pelvic mobility and lower birth hormones, coupled with loss of gravity. The risk is that you are 50% more likely to need an assisted delivery if you have an epidural. Or, if the national average for assisted delivery is 12.9%, with an epidural you have an 18.3% chance of assisted delivery.[61] (See Chapter 19: Assisted Delivery.)

- Due to lowering of birth hormones, there is an increased risk of augmentation of labour (delivery of artificial oxytocin) which has its own set of complications. (See Part 4: Induction of labour.)

- You are more likely to need a caesarean due to foetal distress, however there is no clear link between epidural use and increased overall risk of caesarean.[62]

- The effect of the epidural on hormones can have an effect on breastfeeding as oxytocin and prolactin rates are lower than normal. This may result in more time for milk to come in, and lower volumes of milk being produced at the start.[63]

It is very difficult to get a clear idea on the implications of epidural use, not least because so many other factors are a consideration, such as other pain relief that may have been administered, the specific types of drugs used for epidural, at what point in the labour it is administered, the duration of the administration of the drug, how long the labour has been in progress, the wellbeing of the mother, and other risk factors.

There are plenty of studies that reach conclusions one way or the other, but overall reviews of studies find that clear implications are inconclusive.

What if I do Nothing?

In most cases an epidural is chosen as a last resort for people who have reached the end of their coping mechanism for labour, unless they are having a caesarean section in which case the option to do nothing is usually not possible.

Doing nothing means you need to find other ways to cope with the sensations of labour, getting rest and recuperation in other ways.

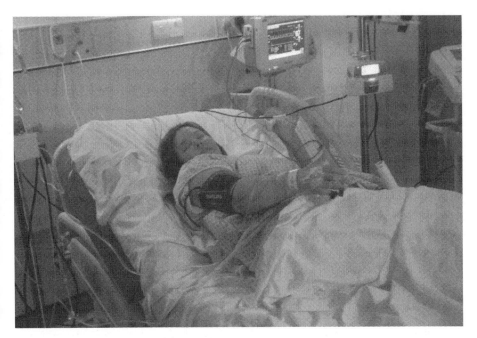

Charlotte lay on her side with her upper body propped up during her epidural to try to keep her pelvis mobile and allow gravity to help her baby move down.

How can I minimise complications?

There are also things that you can do to try to mitigate the negative effects of an epidural. For example, having the mother in a non-supine position – perhaps lying on her side, or even supported on all-fours – would have a huge impact on gravity and pelvic mobility.

Regularly changing the mother's position – lying on one side and switching every 30 minutes or so – can also help the baby move and keep the pelvis semi-mobile.

Studies in the US showed that propping open the mother's legs using a peanut ball (like a gym ball but more peanut-shaped) reduced the rates of caesarean after epidural significantly.[64] While this is a simple technique that could easily be done in any hospital setting, it is relatively new and most hospitals would not even think to do it.

Ways of minimising complications from an epidural include the following.

- Maintain a good birth environment and stay in the zone of labour to help enhance labour hormones – keep lights dim, room quiet, supportive birth partner. It is tempting to just 'switch off from labour' but ultimately this doesn't aid the natural process.

- Rest and re-nourish, and then try to get back into the zone of labour.
- Avoid lying on back, lie on side semi-recumbent (with upper body supported) to help maintain gravity and pelvic mobility.
- Lie on side with leg raised, perhaps using a slightly deflated birth ball or cushions (or anything – your suitcase?) to keep your pelvis open.
- Change which side you are lying on every 30 mins or so (will need help from birth partner and staff) to help maintain pelvic mobility and allow the pelvis and uterus to move around.
- Explore the possibility to lie on front – need plenty of pillows and a supportive team. It is important not to have the belly compressed but being in an all-fours position gives your body the best physiological chance of an unassisted birth.
- Pulling on something (like a rebozo or scarf) may help with pushing.
- Use breathing and visualisations to aid pushing in second stage.

REAL EXPERIENCE: Andrea's Story

It was my first labour and I wasn't sure what to expect but I knew I didn't want a C-section if I could manage without.

My waters broke on a Friday evening, a day before due date in Pizza Express, out for a meal with friends on my husband's birthday. I expected that labour pains and pushing would follow soon and was disappointed to be sent home from hospital midnight Friday night as not much was happening. I struggled to sleep and got very impatient!

By Saturday afternoon I wanted to go back in for reassurance and the contractions had speeded up. We got to the hospital and were told I was 3 cm dilated, if that. I felt so disappointed!

I stayed in and laboured – the midwife left us to wait and walk around. By the evening, they said I could move into midwifery-led room, which was more natural and I assumed I'd soon be meeting our first baby(!) in this room... but things weren't moving quick enough and I was getting tired. So instead I was offered pethidine so I could sleep a bit.

By Sunday morning I was still only 4 cm dilated and they needed to get baby out soon as my waters had broken 36 hours before. So, they mentioned a drip.

To be honest I panicked and burst into tears – I was worried it would mean more and more interventions and my mind jumped to C-section. The midwife was really good and encouraged me to keep going but warned me they'd need to give me an epidural as the contractions would be ramped up as they needed me to deliver in 8 hours. I also needed a catheter – I just went with it all, wanting my baby safe and sound.

Apart from not being able to move around, the drip and epidural did the trick. By 3pm Sunday the midwife allowed the epidural to wear off a bit so I could feel to push – 1 ½hours later my daughter arrived – safe and very alert – the pethidine hadn't affected her.

I needed an episiotomy too. It wasn't as I'd planned at all but the medical staff were brilliant and very encouraging through it all.

REAL EXPERIENCE: *Delyth's Story*

I went to hospital at midnight on Thursday for reduced movement and was told within an hour they would induce me – most of my birth plan now goes out the window!

Pessary was inserted at 2am for 24 hours, and continuous contractions started at 5am. I had pethidine at midday so I could get some sleep,

I was being continuously monitored which was frustrating. The idea that you can move around while being continuously monitored I'd say is pretty much impossible as the straps kept falling off so you're basically confined to the bed.

The pessary was removed at 3am on Saturday but my cervix was still long and hard. Gel was used at 4am and my waters broke naturally at 9am, after which contractions ramped up very quickly.

I was examined at 11am and was still only 1cm dilated. I was moved to labour ward at midday Saturday.

I started using gas and air which pretty much turned me into a lunatic! I found it took about 30 seconds to feel the effect by which point the contraction had finished so I spent any 'downtime' from a contraction in a state of complete panic and spinning out, hallucinating and feeling sick.

I was examined again at 1pm and was still only 1cm dilated so the midwife suggested an epidural. I didn't want pethidine again as I'd had it the previous day.

The epidural was put in at 1:30pm and I had instant relief. My big fear/concern before was feeling out of control and not being able to feel my legs but it was put in really well and I could still feel and move my entire body (just not feel pain). *I even lifted my own legs before the pushing.*

I had a button to top it up myself and I set an alarm for every 25 mins to top it up.

I was put on a hormone drip to increase contractions and the midwife said she'd check on me in 6 hours. Within 3 hours I was feeling pressure and she checked and I was 5cm. An hour later I said I felt like pushing (I could feel a strong urge almost like I needed a poo). Again, I could feel everything but no pain, she checked and I was 10cm dilated.

I started pushing 30 mins later and could really feel where I should be pushing (pelvic floor exercises 100% worked with this, knowing where to push), and my baby was out within 25 mins, the midwife was very experienced and got me panting at the correct time.

Baby arrived at 18:54. I could feel everything that was going on but still no pain. A slight tear which only required one stitch.

I felt in complete control mentally and physically and so pleased I accepted that version of pain relief as the contraction pain and gas and air made me feel very out of control, especially after days of no sleep and the initial shock of an induction. I had the injection to deliver the placenta, didn't feel anything.

Within an hour, I walked myself to a wheelchair and was back up on the ward. Movement returned very quickly. The catheter was quite uncomfortable and annoying so I asked for it to be removed at midnight. Since birth, pain has been managed with paracetamol and ibuprofen only and I've had no adverse effects to the epidural.

REAL EXPERIENCE: *Lucrezia's Story*

With my first labour my waters broke on my due date. I went into hospital soon after and was given diamorphine as I was in a lot of pain but not dilated. It helped me to rest for 3 or 4 hours.

When I would wake up I would have gas and air. Whilst it made me feel sick to start with, it was a godsend personally. My labour, though, wasn't progressing, and in the meantime my baby had turned back-to-back.

I was given water injections in my back to help with the pain. My hospital was trialling them for the first time and I found it helpful for a short while.

Because my contractions were irregular and I wasn't dilating it was suggested that they augment the labour and in the meantime, give me an epidural.

Thankfully the epidural worked first time and apart from the legs tingling and the awful tights, it was OK.

I needed it topped up frequently and didn't like that I had to wait a long time. I think now you can top it up yourself.

I was in so much pain I don't think I could have coped without an epidural and the brilliant staff too.

On day 3, I was fully dilated but baby got stuck so I was sent to theatre for episiotomy and forceps delivery. I was quite scared of the use of forceps however my baby was in distress and needed to come out as soon as possible. After 3 pushes and the assistance of forceps my baby was born.

REAL EXPERIENCE: *Roberta's Story*

I was an excited, nervous and rather impatient first time mum-to-be with a very long pre-labour. That bit where it certainly feels like painful contractions, but as you haven't hit the magic 4 cm dilated, it's not officially labour.

Twenty-four hours in, and my waters broke with meconium which meant that regardless of how far along I was, I was being admitted and monitored.

My TENS machine experience hadn't been particularly satisfactory, but I have the feeling I wasn't using it very effectively and may have started using it too soon.

Initially I didn't get on very well with the gas and air, but a very persistent midwife was really helpful in getting me to use it effectively and I did find it a big help. Not that it took away the pain, but helped me manage it so that I felt a little more in control during contractions and not at the mercy of it.

The advice I got from the midwife was invaluable and she explained the benefits of having an epidural specifically in context of having syntocin which would ramp up the contractions.

Having previously wanted to avoid an epidural I was happy to accept one given the changing circumstances. It didn't take all the pain away, but it took it down a notch and helped during that waiting period when all you do is dilate slowly.

The epidural wasn't perfect but they deliberately let it run down so that I could have more feeling for pushing.

As it turned out my daughter wasn't quite in the right position and too much time had passed since my waters broke so they recommended a caesarean. I had a swift spinal which made all the pain go away and they got her out healthy and happy.

Part 3

Assessing the Mother and Baby

Interventions go along a sliding scale from gently helping things along, to emergency life-saving treatment. We lump them all into this one category despite some interventions being relatively harmless, and others having quite a big impact on many aspects of labour and birth.

Usually you know if the intervention is an emergency and there is no question that you go with that recommendation. The atmosphere in the room will often change and you will get a clear sense that something needs to be done quickly to help the mother or the baby.

In many cases, though, there is time to discuss and there is rarely a need to hurry for most intervention choices.

Interventions have a variety of purposes: to monitor or assess the state of the baby or mother, to get labour started or help it to move along more quickly, or to assist the baby being born, or placenta delivered.

While assessing the state of the mother, and assisting the baby or placenta to be delivered are fairly straight-forward topics to cover, the process of artificial induction of labour is quite complex. It involves a whole series of stages, some of which can be done in isolation, and not every stage is always included. To this end I have separated induction of labour into its own part and I will discuss each of the stages of this process separately.

Chapter 11
Monitoring: Intermittent and Continuous

What is it?

Monitoring is measuring the baby's heart rate in order to assess its health. The frequency and strength of the heart rate is measured.[65] If the heart rate is too high, low, or erratic it can be a sign that the baby is not receiving enough oxygen via the blood and the baby is thought to be 'distressed' and possibly requires help.

What happens?

Intermittent monitoring

Usually monitoring happens intermittently (at frequent intervals) during labour. Your midwife holds a hand-held Doppler against your abdomen, which she will move around until she can find the baby's heartbeat that is amplified and listened to – this is called Ausculation.[66]

NICE recommends monitoring the mother around every 15 minutes in the active phase of labour and up to every 5 minutes in the second stage. The heart rate is monitored for up to a minute.

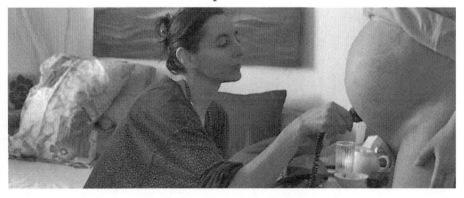

A midwife checks the baby's heartrate at a home birth.

Continuous monitoring

Continuous monitoring is undertaken using electronic equipment known as an electronic foetal monitor (EFM). This can be done externally or internally.

External EFM consists of two sensors strapped to the mother's abdomen – one measures the strength of the contractions, the other measures the baby's heart rate. Movements of the baby and mother can also be captured.

If a good measurement can't be found, internal EFM may be considered. This is where a tiny electrode in the form of a needle is inserted into the scalp of the baby's head through the cervix.

If the baby is considered at risk of hypoxia (lack of oxygen), foetal scalp blood testing may be offered. This is when a tiny blood sample is taken from the baby's scalp in order to determine accurate oxygen levels in the blood.[67]

Both forms of EFM are connected to an electronic device called a cardiotocography (CTG) machine. This can be via wires or wireless depending on the type of machine. This not only monitors the baby's heart rate and mother's contractions, but also keeps a record of it by printing the results onto a long strip of paper. This is known as a trace.

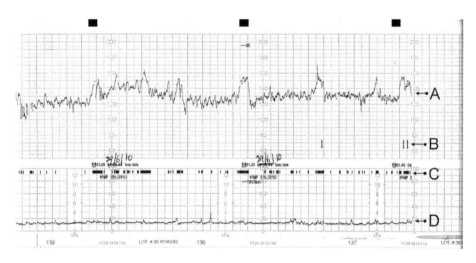

A typical CTG output for a woman not in labour. A: Foetal heartbeat; B: Indicator showing movements felt by mother (caused by pressing a button); C: Foetal movement; D: Uterine contractions

What does it feel like?

Monitoring with a hand-held Doppler is as simple as having a small cylinder, around 3cm in diameter applied with a small degree of pressure to your belly. They are usually wireless and so can be applied to your belly in many positions while you are in labour – often you hardly notice that this is being done.

Continuous foetal monitoring is slightly more invasive insofar as you have two larger monitors – about the size of the palm of your hand – attached to an elasticated strap that is affixed around your body. The elasticated strap needs to be quite tight but it should not be uncomfortable. [68]

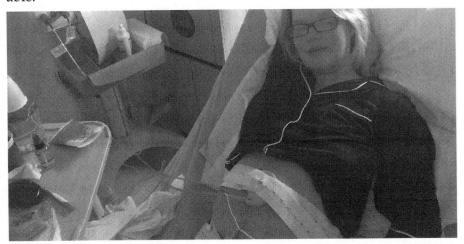

Delyth had foetal monitoring to check the heartrate of her baby.

When is it used?

When you are admitted to hospital you will usually be monitored to achieve a baseline trace – a level to which future heart rates and contraction rates can be compared.

This is done over a 20-minute period, although if you have no indications for the need for monitoring and labour is progressing with no issues then a long monitoring session may well be omitted.

It is then used intermittently during labour to keep an eye on the baby's wellbeing, unless certain interventions or pain relief options are being used which means that continuous monitoring is recommended. These include: use of opioid drugs, epidural, and induction of labour using an oxytocin drip, and is usually recommended with a vaginal birth after caesarean (VBAC).

There may be other medical reasons why continuous monitoring is recommended, and if a hand-held Doppler indicates foetal distress, continuous monitoring is likely to be applied.

NICE guidelines[69] state that continuous monitoring should only be necessary in cases of:

- suspicion of infection or sepsis
- severe Hypotension
- oxytocin use (induction)
- presence of severe meconium
- fresh vaginal bleeding
- high maternal temperature
- high maternal heart rate.

When is it not used?

- You can't have continuous foetal monitoring in a pool, although handheld Dopplers usually have waterproof sheaths so intermittent monitoring can take place.
- You can't have internal monitoring if your membranes are intact.
- You shouldn't have internal monitoring if there are any reasons why vaginal examinations are contraindicated (such as placenta praevia).

What are the Benefits?

The obvious benefit is that the wellbeing of the baby can be closely monitored for signs of 'distress'.

It is also possible with EFM that the strength and intensity of the mother's contractions can also be assessed, and therefore the impact of each contraction on the baby. This can provide reassurance that the baby is ok, and gives us an indication of possible hypoxia (lack of oxygen) identifying whether the baby needs further assistance.

What are the Risks?

EFM can result in restrictions to the mother's movements – she will need to be within a certain distance from the CTG (either dictated by length of wires or wireless range).

If the monitor keeps losing track of the heart rate, the mother may also be encouraged to keep still, possibly lying down on the bed to maximise the machine's ability to pick up the heart rate.

Having continuous foetal monitoring can also cause the mother to divert her attention away from labour, either through being uncomfortable, through having movement restricted which goes against her natural instincts to move or get into a particular position, or through worrying about what the monitor readings are.

There is a controversial debate about the use of continuous foetal monitoring (as opposed to intermittent) in labour as some studies have shown a slight increase in risk of assisted deliveries (14.8% instead of 12.9% national rate) and a significant increase in the risk of caesarean sections (42% instead of national rate of 26.2%) with their use.[70]

The foetal heart rate only shows one picture and this is open to interpretation. Just because a baby's heart rate is variable does not necessarily mean there is a problem and it is not a diagnostic tool in itself. There is also a reliance on the technology being accurate.

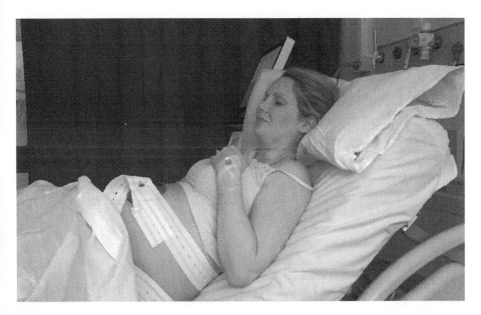

Siobhan was monitored and also had a cannula inserted in case she required the use of remfentanil as she was contraindicated for pethidine or epidural.

Are there any Alternatives?

There are no other ways of monitoring a baby, apart from a traditional stethoscope (it is very hard to pick up the baby's heartbeat with a stethoscope), or an ultrasound which is not commonly used in labour, and is a much more complicated process.

Intermittent monitoring is a very good alternative to continuous monitoring.

What is in question is how useful continuous monitoring is as there is a clear link between continuous foetal monitoring and increased risk of intervention, and very little evidence to show that there are any clear benefits.[71]

What are the Implications?

- In order for the monitor to pick up the baby's heart rate, it has to be in a specific position and if you or your baby move then it can lose the heart rate and need to be repositioned. This can result in the movement of the mother being restricted in order to maintain the trace.

- There is a risk that both the care provider (doctor or midwife) pays more attention to the monitor than the mother, and does not see it as part of the bigger picture.

- The electronic foetal monitor can be distracting in terms of watching the trace and also the sound of the heart rate beeping.

- Movement with continuous foetal monitoring is often restricted, although you can sit, stand, be on ball, etc.

- You may end up being left with a monitor on for longer than planned due to staff attending other people, rather than coming back every 15 minutes as would be required for intermittent monitoring.[72]

- While the heart rate for the baby is constantly monitored, the care provider will not be constantly watching the trace, thus indicating that if a sudden change did occur, they wouldn't be in the room to observe and act upon it anyway.

- You are unable to use a bath, shower or birth pool while being continuously monitored.

- If the external monitor keeps losing the trace, internal monitoring may be used.

- You may have your membranes (waters) broken in order to place the electrode if internal monitoring is chosen.

- To have internal monitoring, the electrode is inserted via the vagina and insertion may be uncomfortable or painful, particularly during contractions.

- Foetal Scalp blood testing may be offered in the case of internal monitoring.

What if I do Nothing?

There is a strong case for not doing continuous foetal monitoring as it doesn't yield clear positive results and can often lead to further intervention.

There is absolutely a choice to decline continuous foetal monitoring, however most people find if there is a concern about the baby then the peace of mind it offers outweighs the cons.

If you are having an induction of labour or epidural, then you won't have a choice about continuous foetal monitoring.

How can I minimise complications?

- Try to use intermittent monitoring for as long as possible.

- Try changing position and measuring heartbeat afterwards to see if the heart rate has improved.

- Switch the sound of the machines off and turn them away from you.

- Ask to have continuous monitoring for a certain time – for example 20 minutes – and then remove the EFM afterwards if baby's heart rate is ok.

- Keep asking for the EFM to be removed if the trace is normal.

- Remain upright and mobile just within a small radius – make smaller movements but keep gravity and pelvic mobility a priority. Sitting on a ball is a good compromise.

- Large movement can make the monitor lose connection with the heart rate – you can always hold it in place, or get your partner to do so.

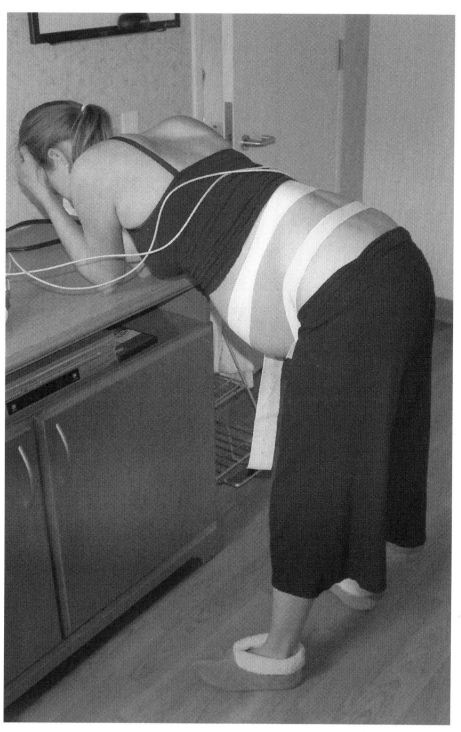

Staying upright is possible with continuous monitoring.

REAL EXPERIENCE: Tanya's Story

I went in [to hospital] due to reduced movements. I was sent home and told to monitor his movements, if he hadn't moved a certain amount of times in a time period to go back.

I went back in the mid-morning and was put on a drip as I was dehydrated. They did struggle to find a vein to add the cannula so ended up with 5 attempt marks on my arm!

Once I was moved to the labour ward they broke my waters and had to put a clip on my son's head to monitor him. The midwife was unable to get the clip on the first time, so the head midwife tried but the second clip broke and on the 3rd time they finally got it on. That was really painful.

By the morning, I was not dilating quickly enough so they decided the best course of action was to have an emergency C-section.

They then added an epidural. The problem is that I get very nauseous when I have anaesthetic. When I was taken into the theatre, I was being physically sick. My whole body was shaking and the anaesthetist was giving me various anti-nausea medicines. I remember the surgeon telling him to keep me still but nothing was working. My son was born not that long after that. Thankfully healthy and with no problems.

REAL EXPERIENCE: Macey's Story

Eva had stopped moving the weekend before she was due, the only movements I felt were of her having hiccups, yet I was still having painless but breathless contractions every 15 minutes.

I ended up ringing the triage around 6pm and they told me to come in to be examined. They hooked me up to the ECG machine from 6.30pm–8.30pm and gave me a button to press every time I felt movement. I think there were only five or six light kicks so the doctor in charge suggested the induction. This same doctor later changed their mind and told me to come back on my due date. I explained how worried I was and the midwife asked the new doctor from the staff change over. The new doctor and the consultant who just happened to be there both agreed to the induction.

After a couple of hours of waiting, they got a junior nurse to do a scan to make sure Eva was in the right position and they did an internal examination to see if I was dilated and it turned out I was 1cm dilated!

At 11pm I was induced and moved to a ward. The next day (Sunday 20th) contractions had kicked in at around 10am.

I told a midwife I couldn't feel Eva move again so she put me on the ECG machine for a couple of hours. Afterwards, I got worried by a stinging sensation in my cervix (never knew it was my cervix dilating!)

The midwife came back with a student midwife and they asked permission if the student midwife could do an internal examination and I agreed. The student midwife couldn't check properly as the pessary was in the way so the proper midwife did the examination and I had dilated another cm.

After a long day of being stuck in the ward with contractions, Jeff came to hospital straight after work around 6pm, and by this point my contractions were two minutes apart.

Three hours later (22 hours after being induced) they brought me down to the delivery unit. I had to be hooked up the ECG machine again (this was on for seven hours) meaning I couldn't move about as easily I wanted, and I couldn't have the water birth as I had planned.

I had to have my waters broken and because my cervix was not facing forward, the midwife had to intervene. After that and being hooked on to the drip the contractions got more and more intense so I started using the gas and air which helped a lot.

When I got to around 5cm dilated, I felt a strong urge to push that I just could not control so the midwife asked me if I wanted diamorphine and I agreed. It knocked me out so much that I was only in so much pain at the peak of each contraction.

Seven hours of contractions went by and I was finally ready. I was pushing for about an hour, there was still the effects of the pain relief which made me feel like I couldn't get into an upright position to make it easier.

After the hour of pushing the midwife asked if I wanted any assistance so I said yes and I agreed to the episiotomy and a ventouse, and within 40 minutes Eva was born and we decided on the injection to deliver the placenta so it was over and done with.

REAL EXPERIENCE: *Fabienne's Story*

When I had my first child, it was an induction after 15 days in hospital due to pre-eclampsia. I had an immediate epidural to try to bring down my blood pressure. Because I had pre-eclampsia, I had continuous monitoring which picked up that the baby's heartbeat was dropping to 48bpm with each contraction and this labour resulted in an emergency C-section.

When I had a VBAC with my second birth, I refused continuous monitoring as I wanted to be able to move around.

The midwives were ok with it at first, but when the baby's heartbeat dropped with each contraction (not as much as with first baby) they insisted I had continuous monitoring. The midwife said she had to do that otherwise she would be neglecting her duty as a midwife.

In the end, I had a successful vaginal birth on gas and air. I did manage a third-degree tear though and had to spend an hour and a half in theatre.

With baby number 3, I made sure that I stood up for most of it. I had continuous monitoring, but the midwife made sure I was happy and comfy and adjusted its position as necessary.

I don't remember it being a massive inconvenience as I was standing up most of the time during labour. I think they may have taken it off when I lay on the bed to give birth.

Chapter 12
Vaginal Examinations

What is it?

A vaginal examination is an internal examination of your cervix and vagina performed by your midwife or doctor. It is used to determine:

- The mother's readiness to go into labour.
- Whether she is in labour or not.
- The progress of labour.
- The position and presentation of the baby.
- The assessment of membranes being broken or not.
- To assess or prevent complications from medical risk factors (such as bleeding, cord prolapse or breech presentation).[73]

The assessment is made through observation of the position of the cervix, its softness, its thickness (effacement), and the amount it is dilated, plus the status of the membranes and baby's position.

A vaginal examination is a way of making a snapshot assessment of one aspect of labour, although there are many other contributing factors to the process of labour (not just the state of the cervix), and gives no indication of how much labour time is left (or how much has elapsed).

What happens?

You will need to get into a reclined or semi-reclined position, with knees bent and open. The midwife or doctor inserts their (gloved) fingers and hand into your vagina and they will use the fingers to feel around the vagina and assess the cervix through touch.

Assessment of cervical dilation is based on the number of fingers that can be entered into the cervix (and could well be argued that it is not particularly 'scientific').

Consent should be obtained before every VE, although in practice some women feel that declining a vaginal examination is not really an option. It is entirely the woman's decision whether to have it at all, and the frequency, although many women feel that they want to try to get a sense of where they are in their labour.

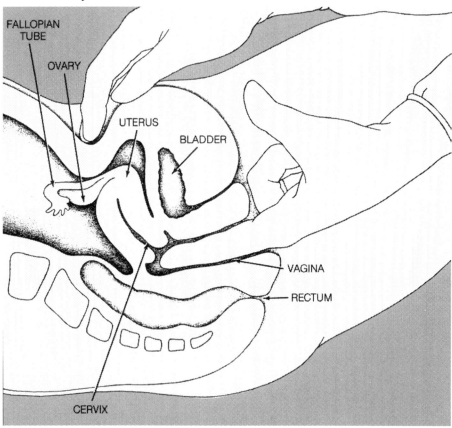

FALLOPIAN TUBE

OVARY

UTERUS

BLADDER

VAGINA

RECTUM

CERVIX

A vaginal examination (outside of pregnancy). Fingers are inserted and the cervix is assessed through judging how far apart the fingers can go which is very subjective. This image shows a non-pregnant body.

When is it used?

A vaginal examination is often given to a woman towards the end of her pregnancy, particularly if she is past 40 weeks in her pregnancy, her estimated due date.

It is also usually offered on arrival to hospital to assess the progress of labour, and this will inform the decision to send the mother back home or admit her.

A vaginal examination is usually offered every 4 hours during labour, following NICE guidelines.[74]

What is confusing is that guidelines state clearly that vaginal examinations should only be conducted when absolutely necessary, and should take the mother's wellbeing and dignity into consideration.

However, they are also considered to be the only way to measure progress of labour (which is not true, and it is also not an accurate measurement[75]) and so they are sometimes offered in such a way as to be felt to be something that cannot be refused.[76] Progress can really only be measured by performing more than one vaginal examination in a period of time as the vaginal examination itself is just a snapshot and can't give any information about how much time has elapsed or will elapse.

There is no evidence to support or reject the use of vaginal examinations in labour as a determinant of labour progress, nor with any difference in outcomes.[77]

When is it not used?

You should not have any vaginal examinations if you have any history of vaginal bleeding, have placenta praevia, have early rupture of membranes (waters breaking) or are in pre-term labour.

You are perfectly within your right to refuse any vaginal examination if you feel uncomfortable for any reason: it is very much a diagnostic tool rather than an intervention as such.

What are the Benefits?

- You get a reasonable sense of how ready you are for labour (before labour starts or how labour is progressing).

- You can get reassurance that labour is progressing, and an idea of the rate of progress.

- You can get a clearer idea of the presentation of the baby.

What are the Risks?

- A vaginal examination could introduce infection, particularly if your waters have broken. This increases with the number of vaginal examinations you have.[78]

- It is not an accurate measurement – using touch to determine a small difference in size is a very subjective yardstick. (Perhaps only 50% accurate.[79])

- Measurement is inconsistent and can differ hugely between different people.[80]
- It can be painful during contractions due to hand position and necessity of reclining.
- It can lead to accidentally rupturing membranes.
- It can feel invasive and undignified.[81]
- It could affect progress of labour, as the emotional state of the mother is delicate and release of stress hormones from a distressing vaginal examination could impact birth hormones and slow down labour.[82]

Are there any Alternatives?

The progress of labour can be assessed largely through the behaviour of the mother. The way she moves, vocalises, what she says, what her emotional state is, the positions she adopts and how able she is to talk and interact both during and in between contractions can give a huge amount of information.

There are also other physiological changes in the mother's body that can be observed without intimacy. A purple line appears on the mother's lower back, from the anal opening up through her buttocks and there is a link between the line and cervical dilation and the position of the baby.

There is also observation of the 'Rhombus of Michaelis', an area encompassing the three lowest lumbar vertebrae, the sacrum and a long ligament that stretches up the back. During the second stage of labour, these bones that form the back wall of the pelvis spontaneously move back, pushing the hip bones further out and making space for the baby.

This can be observed in the lower part of the back, in combination with the mother often reaching her hands up to hold something (thought to help her during this destabilisation of her pelvis). It is oft-observed by midwives but little researched or understood and it comes under the umbrella of 'midwives' wisdom' rather than researched practice, but it is certainly an indicator that could be used as an alternative to a vaginal examination by a midwife experienced in this.[83]

What are the Implications?

- Knowing how dilated you are (or not) can hinder dilation if progress is not as far as expected or hoped.

- By placing your dilation on a chart of 'progress', (or lack thereof), you are placed upon a perceived ideal timeline of labour. Failure to progress along this timeline can result in further interventions such as augmentation of labour, and caesarean.

- It can interrupt labour due to physical touch in a very intimate place. The cervix is quite sensitive to external stimuli and the very act of touching it, could cause it to close up or open more slowly.

- It can interrupt labour due to an emotional reaction influencing a physical one (remember birth is first and foremost a hormonal process and is heavily influenced by the emotional state of the mother).

What if I do Nothing?

Declining vaginal examinations is absolutely an option and there is a lot of evidence to support this decision. Not having a vaginal examination means that you would look to other behaviour of the mother in labour and the picture as a whole to assess progress.

How can I minimise complications?

- Ask if it is really necessary to have a vaginal examination and if you prefer not to then you can decline.

- Ask for less frequent vaginal examinations.

- If you have a vaginal examination, ask for the midwife to wait until you are ready, especially if during labour.

- Avoid vaginal examinations during contractions. Not only can it be uncomfortable, but also you usually have to have a vaginal examination in a reclined position which is less comfortable for labour. Begin the vaginal examination immediately after a contraction so as to aim to have it before the next one starts.

- Ask the midwife to be as quick as possible.

- Ask if the vaginal examination can be performed in non-reclined position.

A good way to prepare for a vaginal examination is to get into the preferred position, lie back, close your eyes and do some deep breathing. With each exhale consciously relax your belly, buttocks and vagina.

When you are ready, let the midwife know. As she conducts the vaginal examination, continue breathing deeply keeping as relaxed as possible. This should minimise discomfort.

REAL EXPERIENCE: Cassie's Story

I went into labour at 5.45am by hearing and feeling my mucous plug pop! Contractions started within 30 mins and were about 20–30 minutes apart for most of the day.

I tried get on with normal life. I went to Co-op and had a contraction in the cheese aisle! Then I made bread!

By the evening the contractions were pretty close together and intensive and so we called for a midwife to check me out and she arrived around 1am (I was having a home birth).

She was so lovely, her name was Nicki I think, and she was kind and chatty. She wanted to do a vaginal exam to check my dilation and I readily agreed as we were so excited about meeting our baby really soon. I felt it was really going to help me be motivated as I was in pain and feeling tired by this point.

I said to her, if I am only 1cm dilated please don't tell me, just lie! Just tell me I'm 2 cm!'. She finished the exam, sat back and said, 'you're 1cm dilated!'

It was a massive blow! We had really thought we were near the end but it hadn't even really started. She suggested having a cry and a glass of wine (which we did – it helped) and then she left us to it.

I had a further 3 midwife visits in the next 48 hours and by the 3rd time (Tuesday early hours) she said I was at that magic 4 cm dilated so she would stay with me and I could finally get into the birth pool.

Sadly, I hated the sensation of being in the water and I was completely exhausted. I transferred to hospital and took gas and air – it was WONDERFUL! I had only had a TENS machine up to that point.

I ended up having quite a lot of interventions and pain relief, but I avoided an epidural and feel very proud of myself for having coped for so long with no pain relief.

REAL EXPERIENCE: Astrid's Story

As a woman, you have a vaginal examination every few years for your pap smear test. In late pregnancy and labour, I had a number of examinations to check my readiness for labour.

They were all different depending on who did them. The first time was quite uncomfortable and unpleasant but then my pregnancy yoga teacher advised me to lie back, and use deep breathing to help relax, and during my exhales to really relax my vagina muscles. This really helped. A LOT!

While it doesn't really feel very dignified, after a few times you don't mind and it was really helpful to get a sense of how close labour or birth were likely to be.

Part 4
Induction of Labour

Induction of labour seems like a simple, single process. In reality it is comprised of a series of interventions that generally happen in a certain order, in order to either stimulate labour to begin (induction) or help it progress more quickly (augmentation).

You can go through part of the induction journey and change your mind, however, after a certain point it is a one-way street and you can't opt out.

As each stage in the induction process is an intervention in itself, I have separated out the whole process into its own part, with each element covered in a separate chapter.

To help understand the entire process I include an overview here, and that is then broken down into its constituent parts.

Before I get into details I think it is useful to talk about the Bishop score, a tool to determine readiness for labour.

Bishop score

Bishop score is a system used to determine the body's 'readiness for labour' and so can give an indication of the likelihood of an induction of labour being successful or not, and therefore whether to proceed or not.

It is a point-scoring system based on the position, consistency and stretchiness of the cervix, how thin (effaced) and open it is (dilated) and the position of the baby's head in relation to the cervix (engaged).[84] The measurements are conducted as part of a vaginal examination.

These five components are assessed and each given a score, and the overall score is then used as a measurement of readiness.

Here is a table that shows the scoring system.[85] Originally the measurements of dilation needed to be specific, although an updated version indicates more flexible measurements.

	Score			
Component	0	1	2	3
Cervical position	Posterior	Middle	Anterior	-
Cervical consistency	Firm	Medium	Soft	-
Effacement	<30%	40–50%	60–70%	>80%
Dilation	Closed	1–2cm	3–4cm	>5cm
Foetal Engagement	-3	-2	-1, 0	+1, +2

The total score possible is 13, and if the score is 8 or above the likelihood of a successful induction is usually considered the same possibility as with spontaneous onset of labour. An induction undertaken with a score of 5 or lower has an increased risk of caesarean.[86]

Cervical position: outside of labour, the cervix is positioned high in the vagina and quite far towards the back of the body (posterior). As the body gets closer to labour the position of the cervix lowers and comes forward (anterior), partly due to the pressure of the baby's head wwagainst it.

Cervical consistency: the cervix outside of labour is usually hard and resistant to stretching in order to maintain integrity and keep the baby inside. In the days leading up to labour the cervix starts to soften to allow effacement and dilation.

Effacement: this is how thick or thin the cervix is. Usually it is around 3–4cm long and about 2–3cm wide. In early labour, the cervix draws back into the uterus becoming thinner and thinner until it is not discernible any longer.

Dilation: this is the opening of the cervix and is a result of the baby's head pressing against it. Once the cervix has fully thinned, it will start to draw back around the baby's head, to full dilation around 10cm in diameter. At this point the baby's head is already almost halfway through the cervix.

Foetal engagement: this is the position of the baby's head in relation to the ischial spines (a bony protrusion) in the pelvis. The ischial spines can't be felt and so this position can only be estimated. It is usually gauged by the midwife palpating the mother's abdomen just above the pubic bone so see how much of the baby's head can be felt.

Nearly all of these methods of measurement are subjective and dependent upon the sensation of touch, and the opinion of the person conducting the examination, and so could, in theory, come out with a different score if undertaken by different people.

The Bishop score is a factor in determining how successful an induction might be but is not always the most effective tool, just like cervical dilation is not a good indicator of relative progress of labour.[87] Nevertheless it is a useful indicator and is commonly used to determine likely outcome of induction.

Chapter 13
Induction of Labour (Overview)

What is it?

An induction is to medically start labour before the mother's body is naturally ready through the application of hormones called prostaglandins (brand name: Propess) to soften cervix, then a drip with artificial oxytocin (Syntocinon) to stimulate contractions.

Success or not is directly related to how 'ripe' the cervix is. An assessment of the cervix is made through a vaginal examination and a points-based system called the Bishop score is used to calculate the 'readiness' of the body to go into labour.

What happens?

There are many stages to an induction. Generally speaking, they go in this order, although depending on the Bishop score, you may find you skip a stage.

1. You are offered a stretch and sweep at 40+ weeks (midwife). This may be repeated a number of times in the next 2 weeks.

2. Induction is discussed and booked in.

3. Arrive at hospital – initial assessment (1–2 hours plus waiting).

   a. Vaginal examination to assess Bishop score.

   b. Monitor the baby's heart rate (continuous foetal monitoring to get base rate), usually for 20 minutes.

   c. Monitor mother's blood pressure, temperature, urine sample taken.

   d. Admit you to the induction ward (if they have space).

4. Prostaglandin pessary (up to 24 hours) to soften cervix, hopefully start contractions and initiate dilation of cervix.

a. Pessary inserted vaginally.

b. Lie down for 30 mins. Then you're allowed to move around and sometimes you can go home.

c. As soon as labour starts, the pessary is removed (24 hours is allowed for pessary to work).

5. Artificial rupture of membranes (up to 2 hours) if cervix is dilated enough to stimulate contractions.

a. Hook inserted into vagina, through cervix to break membranes (waters).

b. This can only be done if you are a little bit dilated.

c. If labour starts naturally then you can opt out of rest of induction, but you can't leave hospital.

6. Oxytocin drip (up to 12–24+ hours) to artificially stimulate labour.

a. Pitocin administered via drip. The drip is not removed once it is in.

b. Contractions start very quickly.

c. You have to be continuously monitored.

d. You will be expected to dilate at 1cm per hour.

e. Once baby is born, you will have active management of the third stage (injection to deliver placenta).

When is it used?

NICE guidelines say the only reasons for an induction are:

• Prolonged pregnancy (anything after 40 weeks, although anytime up to 42 weeks is not technically overdue).

• If your waters have broken but your contractions have not started after 24 hours (76.5% start contractions within 24 hours[88]).

• Medical conditions that result in higher risk of complication or stillbirth, such as gestational diabetes,[89] choleostasis,[90] and IVF.[91]

• Maternal request in exceptional circumstances.

• Stillbirth.

The key reason for offering an induction is because of an increased risk of stillbirth with prolonged pregnancy. The risk of stillbirth doubles between 41–42 weeks. However alarming this might sound, you have to remember the difference between relative risk and absolute risk.

The *actual* risk of a stillbirth, according to NICE, is 2–3 per 1000 births over 40 weeks, and by 42 weeks that number has gone up to 5–6 per 1000.[92]

The *relative* risk has doubled but in real terms this is an increase from 0.3% to 0.6%. These are tiny numbers. You have to induce 500 women to save one baby.

Other reasons that are given for inducing labour include:

- Having a big baby, or a small baby. Bear in mind that scans assessing the size of a baby can be 30% inaccurate when done at 40 weeks, plus it is physiologically possible to give birth to a huge baby with no complications.

- A previous history of shoulder dystocia. This is where the shoulder of the baby gets stuck during delivery. Larger babies are more likely to get stuck, but the position of the mother when giving birth plays a role in this risk as well.[93]

- Reduced movements of the baby indicating possible foetal distress or other issue.[94]

- Reduced or excessive amniotic fluid.[95]

All of these reasons should be considered on a case-by-case basis, and the risks of induction itself should be considered alongside the risk of the reason for induction.

When is it not used?

Induction is not used if the mother has had a previous caesarean. This is due to the increased risk of hyperstimulation of the uterus, and uterine rupture with an induction following a previous caesarean.

Certain medical conditions may also be contraindicated and these are dealt with in the individual chapters below.

What are the Benefits?

These benefits outline the benefits for an induction although specific stages of induction have their own set of benefits and risks. Please refer to the relevant chapters for more information.

- It reduces risk of stillbirth from 0.6% to 0.3% in a pregnancy that has gone past 41 weeks, or more if the risk factors for the mother are higher due to a specific medical condition.

- If waters have broken and labour has not started, it reduces risk of infection.
- The labour itself is generally quicker – this may be beneficial for the mother.
- You have more certainty about when baby will arrive, although the entire process can still take anything from a few hours to many days.

What are the Risks?

- Induction can result in sudden onset of painful and intensive contractions.
- It has an impact on birth hormones that interfere with the natural process and the body's ability to cope with the pain.
- There are side effects of the drugs involved (see Chapter 16: Oxytocin Drip).
- The effects on the baby are not fully understood,[96] and in some studies, have been shown to be detrimental to the baby.[97] This could well be due to the fact that babies are often induced before their due date or before they are naturally ready, indicating that they are in some respects under-developed.[98]

In my own Active Birth teacher training in March 2014, Janet Balaskas said that, 'Induction is the most predictable way to create an abnormal labour and a need for operative delivery.'

Are there any Alternatives?

Be patient! There have been studies that have discovered that when a baby's lungs are fully developed (and ready to start breathing air at maximum efficiency outside the uterus), a protein is released in the lungs that activate two genes. This results in an inflammatory response from the mother that triggers labour: essentially babies are born when they are ready.[99]

If you just have a prolonged pregnancy (are overdue) – you can be monitored daily by hospital to ensure the wellbeing of baby and mum. This is known as expectant management. It usually involves going to hospital and having a period of continuous foetal monitoring, plus an assessment of the mother (blood pressure, urine sample, etc.).

If your waters have broken, you can have antibiotics to help avoid risk of infection.

There are a variety of natural methods to enhance labour. These usually concentrate on increasing the mother's oxytocin levels, and creating an environment for the birth hormones to thrive.

There are various foods, herbs and therapies said to help naturally induce labour,[100] however if they were really that efficacious then we would not need a medical induction!

What are the Implications?

The implications across each part of an induction vary, but overall:

- You are often restricted in location – inductions are performed on a delivery suite only.
- You are restricted in terms of movement and positions.
- You will need continuous foetal monitoring.
- You are more likely to require pain relief,[101] and using certain pain relief options have further implications for intervention.
- There is a risk of baby being distressed due to intensity of labour, this could lead to further intervention.
- You can't use a birth pool or get in the shower.
- You are more likely to require assistance for birth,[102] however this is influenced by other pain relief options chosen.
- Active management of the third stage is required.

What if I do Nothing?

Being patient and doing nothing is very much encouraged if there is no clear medical reason for performing an induction. The great thing is that you can reassess each day and change your mind about doing nothing if you have any concern about your baby.

Seventy percent of babies come within 10 days of their due date and so being patient and trusting your body can often lead to spontaneous onset of labour.

If you are looking at an induction due to medical reasons then the risk of doing nothing should be taken into consideration on a case-by-case basis.

How can I minimise complications?

- Make sure that your decision to undertake an induction is with full understanding of the medical reasons. Ask for statistics and an explanation of the absolute risks if necessary.
- Ask for a low dose of oxytocin to be administered to start with.
- Keep upright and mobile to assist the natural movement of the baby.
- Keep an appropriate birth environment to help natural hormones flow.
- Do as much birth preparation as possible to have plenty of tools to help cope with the sensations of labour.
- Try to avoid pain relief, particularly epidural.
- Experience as much skin-to-skin, eye contact and breastfeeding after birth as possible – this helps hormones balance and get back to normal.

REAL EXPERIENCE: Katie's Story

I had gestational diabetes and was told I would have to be induced early. I was examined and had the first pessary inserted by 7.30 Thursday morning. I was admitted on to a ward for monitoring but told they would come around every 4 hours to check baby's heartbeat.

In between I was advised to walk around/use a birthing ball to help things along (which I did.) I was examined the following morning – this was always agony because of my pelvic pain – then they inserted a second pessary.

I walked around the hospital again all day and could start to feel mild contractions. These gradually got stronger throughout the day.

At about 6pm when they checked baby's heartbeat, she kept moving around and the nurse became worried that she was in distress. I was suddenly rushed down to a delivery suite in a big panic, which really scared me!

They calmed me down and managed to find baby's heartbeat which had returned to a normal rate – they said it was probably just that she was trying to get away from being poked and prodded and worked herself up.

After being monitored for quite a while I was taken back up to the ward and everything had slowed right down. At least this meant I was able to have a good night's sleep.

I was examined again mid-morning on Saturday and was told I was just dilated enough to have my waters manually ruptured. The midwife took a good 10 minutes explaining to me how long I could be waiting to go down to delivery (2 days or more!) however just as she finished talking, a nurse came in to take me down there and then!

In the delivery suite, there was a minimum of 1 person with me at all times and I had the monitoring belt on at all times too. My waters were ruptured and the synthetic hormone drip started; this was gradually increased at equally spaced intervals.

We hit another road bump early evening when they kept losing baby's heartbeat again (because she was moving so much.) The drip was stopped until they could continually see it – this was attempted by attaching a monitoring probe to her head, which was horrendously painful and was eventually given up on in favour of returning to the belt.

When they could establish a regular heartbeat again the drip was started back from where it was stopped – this meant a sudden, massive increase in my contractions/the pain.

I believe it was around this point that they asked if I would like a diamorphine injection to help with the pain, which was gratefully accepted! Up until that point I had just had gas and air.

By 9pm that Saturday I felt the need to start pushing – the midwife told me it was probably just the position of baby because I was only about 5cm the last time they examined me, but she'd examine me again just to check.

Surprisingly I had got to 9cm dilated in a very short space of time. From there it took an hour and a half until Isla was born.

I was there for nearly a further 2 hours to deliver the placenta – I was told they were minutes away from taking me into theatre to remove it. Baby happy and healthy weighing 7 pounds 10.5.

REAL EXPERIENCE: Lisa's Story

Due to prolonged rupture of membranes and group B strep, I was induced to start labour. My contractions came pretty thick and fast (hyper-contracting, I think they called it) and it wasn't long before I needed gas and air, quickly followed by an epidural.

The epidural failed so I carried on with the gas and air (I found a great help with breathing deeply). My baby ended up getting stuck so I was taking to theatre for a forceps delivery, and at this point they gave me a spinal.

My baby's heart rate dropped as soon as the forceps were placed on his head so I ended up having an emergency C-section.

My little boy was born weighing a whopping 10lb 10oz (and I am very small) so it's no wonder he got 'stuck'. He wasn't well after birth and was taking off to NICU before I got to hold him. He is now a bouncing 5-year-old though!

I went on to have a second son via an elective C-section. I had grand plans for my first delivery which I managed to achieve none of. The second time around I just wanted to hold my baby when he was born. My wish came true and I couldn't have asked for a more perfect delivery!

Chapter 14
Membrane Sweep

What is it?

A membrane sweep (also known as a stretch and sweep) is a manipulation of the membranes surrounding the baby in order to stimulate labour to begin.

The membranes inside the cervix are separated from the uterus wall, and this is designed to stimulate a natural release of prostaglandins which increases the likelihood of labour starting spontaneously.

What happens?

Your midwife will ask you to lie down on a couch, naked from the waist down, with knees bent and legs open.

She will insert a gloved hand into your vagina, insert one finger into the cervix and 'sweep' it around in a circular fashion, to separate the membranes from the uterus wall. She may also massage the cervix to help it ripen for labour.[103]

When is it used?

A membrane sweep is usually the first port of call for women who are looking at an induction, particularly for post-dates (i.e., going over your due date).

It is offered by your midwife from 39 weeks in order to encourage labour to start naturally and to avoid an induction.

It can be done as many times as you wish, and can be done at home, in the GP surgery or in any midwife appointment.

While it is not really considered to be part of the induction process by most women, it is nevertheless a mechanical intervention (as opposed to a chemical one) and is an indication of impatience or implication that the mother's body is not 'working correctly' (i.e., going into labour 'on time').[104]

When is it not used?

A membrane sweep is not used in the following cases.

- Placenta praevia or low lying placenta.
- Undiagnosed bleeding in pregnancy.
- Unengaged position of baby.
- Breech or transverse presentation.
- Very large baby.[105]
- Closed and hard cervix.

What are the Benefits?

The main benefit of a membrane sweep is that it encourages labour to begin without recourse to further intervention.[106]

While the membrane sweep in itself is an intervention, most women prefer to attempt this invasive, yet fairly safe intervention in order to avoid the use of hormones or artificial rupture of membranes.

- It can be done in any setting and does not require admission to hospital.
- It can be repeated as many times as is deemed necessary.
- There are no drugs involved and so does not affect the hormones of labour adversely.
- It does not have an effect on the baby.

What are the Risks?

The side effects of a membrane sweep are minimal and are usually an indication that it might be working. These include:

- Discomfort or pain during the procedure.
- Discharge or mild spotting.
- Mild to severe cramps.

There are also some risks including accidental rupture of membranes. While this is not exactly a complication (and is one of the stages of an induction), it increases the chances of infection and set you on the 24hour clock of needing to go into labour naturally (see Chapter 15: Artificial rupture of membranes).[107]

In some cases, you can also have mild to severe bleeding which could result in admission to hospital for treatment or possible induction, or in severe cases, a caesarean.

There is also a risk that bacteria could be introduced to the uterus causing an infection.

One of the key criticisms for it is that it often does not work and different studies have shown that it is both effective and no different than waiting.[108] It seems to be most effective for women at 40–41 weeks of pregnancy with a high Bishop score, however this rather begs the question that perhaps they were just ready to go into labour anyway.

Are there any Alternatives?

The main alternative for membrane sweeping is to be patient!

What are the Implications?

Implications for this procedure are not set in stone. It seems that you are less likely to need a formal induction (for every seven membrane sweeps, one woman avoids an induction).[109]

However, by choosing a membrane sweep it gives the impression that the body is not working correctly and that implies that if the sweep 'does not work' then further intervention may be deemed necessary.

What if I do Nothing?

Patience is the only sure fire way to ensure your baby is born. Doing nothing is absolutely an option and you can change your mind at any point about having a sweep later.

What can I do to minimize complications?

Similar techniques as for having a vaginal examination can be used, after all it is similar to a vaginal examination with a bit more involvement.

Adopting a comfortable position, asking to wait until you are ready, plus spending a few moments to breathe deeply and relax your lower body can really help to reduce discomfort.

REAL EXPERIENCE: Elle's Story

My first baby was very late, big and I had a long and hard labour ending in complications. For my second baby I was advised to have an induction at 40 weeks and knew I wanted to avoid it if at all possible.

Midwives often offer a sweep at 40 weeks but I persuaded my midwife to give me one at 39+5. She did it at my appointment in the GP surgery. The usual strip off lower half and lie on couch with legs akimbo (bent knees, falling outwards). She lubed up her gloved hand and gently inserted her fingers into my vagina.

I was given advice to be as relaxed as possible so I lay back, closed my eyes and just did really deep breaths and consciously relaxed every part of my body.

The sweep was slightly uncomfortable – about the same level as a cervical smear without the scrape. It was done very quickly. Sadly, it didn't do ANYTHING!

I ended up having another 3 sweeps over the next 10 days – and the most painful was done by a small male consultant in the hospital. You would expect someone with small hands to be the best but actually it was quite vigorous and painful that time – perhaps having it done by a man didn't really help me relax.

In the end, I had my waters broken and that was enough to get labour to start so I did avoid the oxytocin drip and had a fantastic quick and easy labour.

Chapter 15
Prostaglandin Gel or Pessary

What is it?

Prostaglandin or dinoprostone[110] is a hormone which aids in the ripening of the cervix in readiness for labour, and can stimulate uterine contractions to induce labour.[111]

It comes in two forms, a gel (brand name Prostin) or a slow-release pessary (brand name Propess[112]).

What happens?

In a reclined position, the gel suppository or pessary is inserted by hand into the vagina to sit next to the cervix. The pessary has a string that is left hanging from the vagina – much like a tampon – and so it can be removed easily.

The hormone from the pessary is slowly released at the cervix over a period of 24 hours.

If gel is used, a second dose may be inserted into the vagina after 6–8 hours if labour has not started.

The dosage and number of treatments will vary depending on the drugs used and hospital policy.

Depending on the hospital policy you may be allowed home until signs of labour begin, at which point you are advised to return to hospital for assessment. You may be asked to stay at hospital and will be admitted onto a ward.

When is it used?

Prostaglandin is used as the first stage of an induction of labour, when the cervix is considered 'unfavourable' (Bishop score of less than 5).

Indications for using a prostaglandin are one or more of the following:

- Cervix is high in the vagina in posterior position.
- Cervix is hard, thick and not dilated at all.
- Baby is high in the pelvis.

It can sometimes be the only trigger the body needs to go into labour naturally. If contractions occur with prostaglandins then further intervention may not be necessary.

When is it not used?

Prostaglandin is not used for the following reasons.

- If the baby has an unusually large head, or is in a sub-optimal position for labour.
- Previous surgery or rupture of the uterus.
- Placenta Praevia.
- Unexplained vaginal bleeding.
- Previous caesarean.
- Allergy to the drug.
- If your waters have broken.[113]
- Contractions have started.
- Foetal distress.
- Increased risks due to medical contraindications such as asthma, glaucoma, liver or kidney disease, and other pregnancy complications (your midwife will consider these before administering the drug).

It would also not be used if your cervix is in the early stages of dilation, as this stage would probably then be skipped in favour of artificially rupturing the membranes.

What are the Benefits?

The benefits of using a prostaglandin are:

- Helping cervix to ripen, and encouraging the body to go into labour naturally.
- If labour starts with prostaglandin, further intervention can be avoided.

- Around 60% of women have their babies within 24 hours of having the prostaglandin.[114]
- You can change your mind about having the prostaglandin and have the pessary removed or decline further intervention.
- You can begin the process of inducing labour for medical reasons and thus starting to reduce the risk to the mother or baby.
- Likelihood of caesarean with just prostaglandin use is reduced (compared with full induction).[115]

What are the Risks?

Side effects of the drugs include:

- Nausea, vomiting and diarrhoea.
- Distress to the baby due to intensive contractions.
- Uterine rupture (very rare).
- Blood clotting issues (very rare).
- Anaphylactic (allergic) reaction (very rare).

As with all drugs, the full list of side effects is long and range from mild to severe. It is advisable to get a full list from your midwife, or look at the documentation of the drugs.

Are there any Alternatives?

There are alternatives to using a prostaglandin but they tend to be out of favour in current obstetric practice.

Use of a Foley catheter is thought to be as effective as prostaglandins but has fewer side effects. A Foley catheter is a thin tube with a balloon that is inserted into the cervix and inflated with fluid in order to start dilating the cervix and stimulate contractions.[116] Once the cervix has dilated sufficiently the catheter drops out.

It stimulates cervical dilation through pressure akin to the baby's head pressing on the cervix.

As it is a mechanical rather than hormonal method, it doesn't have any of the side effects associated with prostaglandin use, although overall length of labour tended to be higher.[117]

There are no equivalent drugs and while natural prostaglandin stimulation through manual stimulation of the cervix could be considered, there is no clear evidence to suggest an appropriate way to do this.

What are the Implications?

Use of the gel rather than pessary necessitates a higher number of vaginal examinations in order to insert the gel numerous times.

There is evidence that if the prostaglandins don't work after long or repeated use, then the likelihood of the induction to fail and result in caesarean section increases.[118]

What if I do Nothing?

At the point of using prostaglandin, you have usually already chosen to undergo an induction of labour. This is the first step in this process so doing nothing implies that you are not ready to start the process.

You can absolutely do nothing, just make sure that if there are any medical reasons for doing an induction that you balance the risks to you or your baby.

What can I do to minimise complications?

- Ask for a pessary so you can minimize vaginal examinations.
- Ask to be allowed to go home so you can generate an appropriate birth environment to encourage the body's natural hormones to work.

REAL EXPERIENCE: Jo's Story

After meticulously planning a home birth without intervention, my birth story was nothing like I could have imagined, but looking back, wonderful nonetheless.

I was induced with a pessary at 8am and by 10am I was having extremely strong contractions with no gaps. The pain was intense, like period pain but sharper, however it was manageable and I breathed through it for about 6 hours.

I then requested some gas and air when they got a bit stronger, which really helped. It doesn't take the pain away, it just makes you feel more relaxed and a little less focused on the pain.

Also, the process of breathing the gas and air gave something to focus the mind on which helped a lot.

By about 8pm I was struggling to manage strong cramps, which were so close together I was getting tired. I was offered some diamorphine which worked quickly and made me much less aware of the discomfort I was in. I remember having a couple of quite relaxed hours after that, where I was able to manage the contractions with a small amount of effort.

Diamorphine just makes you feel really fuzzy and warm, but still 'with it' enough to have sensible conversations with those around you. When the diamorphine wore off at about midnight, was when I began to need something more.

Labour was not progressing and the next step was the hormone drip, and I requested an epidural. I do remember feeling extremely uncomfortable at this point and the pain was not manageable for me. It did not feel like a natural pain, but much sharper.

This did not last for long, because as soon as the epidural was administered, there was no more pain. I got some rest.

Through the night, the hormone drip was turned on and off as it was affecting my baby's heart rate and I was not progressing so at 7.30am I was taken down for an emergency caesarean.

Although C-section had been the last thing on my mind, I

was relieved to have an end in sight. Due to complications with baby's heart rate I didn't have much time to think about it and we went to theatre.

I was extremely nervous about the C-section. I was convinced I would feel everything and I was a bit panicked. The staff could not have been more reassuring and the anaesthetist held my hand through the whole procedure.

All I could feel was a little painless tugging and my little boy arrived shortly after, healthy and noisy!

After coming home I was upset that I didn't have control over my labour and this played on my mind for a while but this slowly ebbed away and I look back on the experience with happy emotions.

However, I firmly believe that in my case, the induction was what caused the complications I had, and next time I will let my body go into labour when it is ready. I am pregnant again now, so I am looking forward to putting this into practice soon :)

Chapter 16
Artificial Rupture of Membranes (Amniotomy)

What is it?

Artificial rupture of the membranes, or amniotomy, is a technique that uses a sharp tool to pierce the amniotic sac to 'break the waters'. This can speed up labour due to the increased pressure of the baby's head onto the cervix that stimulates birth hormones.[119]

In a process of induction, it can also be used as a method to initiate the onset of labour, either after or instead of prostaglandins.

What happens?

You are required to lie in a reclined position, similar to that for a vaginal examination.

Your midwife will insert either an amniocot (a special glove with a sharp point on one of the fingertips), or an amniohook (a long thin implement with a hook on the end) into the vagina, through the cervix and will use the sharp end to pierce the amniotic sac.

This results in the amniotic fluid leaking out through the vagina and increases the pressure of the baby's head onto the cervix.

When is it used?

Artificial rupture of membranes is used as part of the process of induction, in order to help initiate the onset of labour. This can be done on its own, with time left to see if labour starts spontaneously (you may need to request this), but is usually followed immediately by an oxytocin drip.

It can also be used in order to monitor the state of the amniotic fluid if there is some concern that the baby is distressed (meconium in the water can indicate foetal distress).

If the decision has been made to use internal foetal monitoring, the water may be broken to allow the needle to be placed into the baby's scalp.

If labour is felt to be stalling then artificial rupture of membranes can be used to help the labour progress.

When is it not used?

Artificial rupture of the membranes is not used in the following instances.

- If you have vasa previa, a condition where the baby's blood vessels run close to the cervix.[120]

- If vaginal delivery is not planned.

- If the baby appears to be breech or transverse in presentation.

What are the Benefits?

The benefits of artificial rupture of membranes stem from two areas: the intention to speed up labour, and the intention to avoid further intervention (i.e., oxytocin drip and caesarean).

Artificial rupture of membranes can be effective at causing labour to start spontaneously, and can help to progress a stalled or long labour. The actual effectiveness is difficult to measure but is thought to only shorten labour by 60–120 minutes which is not that big a difference in the grand scheme of labour (that can last some days), and some studies reveal no clear change in length of labour; the real benefit here is a contentious subject.[121]

The benefits of this seem closely linked to the point in labour that the membranes are ruptured, but again there is no clear idea as to the optimal time to do so.

This intervention, in turn, helps the mother avoid having to have an oxytocin drip to initiate labour, and also perhaps to augment her labour (when oxytocin is administered after labour has started).[122]

Another benefit is being able to place an internal monitor onto the baby's scalp if there is concern about the baby, and this could help to avoid a caesarean.

It also can give an indication of the state of the amniotic fluid which could give an indication of the baby's wellbeing.

There have been studies that show a link between early artificial rupture of membranes and improvement in the baby's wellbeing at birth.

There have also been studies that look at the reduction in risk of dystocia (where the baby's shoulders get stuck during delivery).[123]

What are the Risks?

The risks associated with artificial rupture of membranes are:

- Discomfort during the procedure.

- The possibility of cord compression or prolapse (where the cord gets stuck between the baby's head and the cervix and could potentially cut off the baby's blood supply) is increased, particularly if the head is not fully engaged. One study puts this risk at 1 in 300.[124]

- Risk of bleeding.

- Risk of slight injury to baby's head (if the hook used catches the baby).

- Increased pain of labour.

- Increased risk of infection.

Are there any Alternatives?

As this is a direct physical intervention onto the birthing process, there is no real alternative. If artificial rupture of membranes is recommended to initiate labour, then a membrane sweep could be an alternative but often by this point the mother may have had more than one sweep already and it has proved thus far to be ineffective.

The idea is that the artificial rupture of membranes helps to increase oxytocin levels in the mother which then helps labour progress. There are many benign ways of stimulating oxytocin that could be just as effective, even in the cases of initiating labour. For example, upright position of mother; dark, warm and private room; support of birth partner; hugs and kisses from birth partner; and use of a birth pool (in established labour – this also has the advantage of pain relief).[125]

The main alternative is to be patient and allow the labour to progress spontaneously.

What are the Implications?

- Increased pain may result in requiring pain relief where none was required before.

- If the amniotic fluid showed signs of meconium (baby's poo) in them, this could lead to further interventions.

- The risk of caesarean increases with artificial rupture of membranes.

- It may have no discernible effect but as an intervention has been performed to assist labour to 'progress', this may be seen as a failure and further intervention may be recommended.

What can I do to minimise complications?

- Try to be really calm and relaxed during the procedure (see Chapter 11: Vaginal Examinations).

- Follow advice on reducing risk of infection for example, do not insert anything into the vagina.

- Take other measures to increase oxytocin levels, and use gravity to help labour progress.

- Request a few hours before oxytocin is administered in order to encourage the spontaneous onset of labour (this is often enough with subsequent labours to get things going).

REAL EXPERIENCE: Kiera's Story

I was told I needed to have an induction at 40 weeks as my first baby was very large and so my first labour was very long and drawn out and ended up with an epidural and forceps delivery due to shoulder dystocia (where the baby's head is born but the shoulder gets stuck).

I was adamant I didn't want an induction and luckily every consultant I saw as my due date got closer had a different story and in the end I was reluctantly booked in for an induction at 40+12. On the one hand, I REALLY didn't want an induction, but on the other hand I was so fed up of being pregnant that my emotions were all over the place.

We turned up on Thursday morning at 8am as planned and spent about 1.5 hours being assessed – about 30 minutes on a monitor to get a baseline reading, urine tests, blood pressure, and a vaginal examination to assess my Bishop score (was on the borderline of successful induction). They also gave me a sweep for good measure as I was already 2cm dilated, and this also meant I wouldn't need the pessary.

We then had to hang around in a waiting room to wait for a room to be available and by about 1pm they told us to go home! So, having an induction wasn't such an emergency then was it!!! It was pretty disappointing having psyched ourselves up for it only to be sent home.

They phoned us at 9pm that night and told us to come in which I refused to do on the ground of it being 9pm at night! The midwife was pretty rude and indicated that 'some people would feel lucky and they might not have space for us in the morning'!

We said we'd take that chance and get a good night's sleep. We called first thing on Friday morning and were told to come in at 1pm. By 4pm we had been admitted and given a room.

I had been advised by a consultant during my pregnancy that I could try to break my water to kick-start labour and wait for 2 hours before going on a drip. I had to fight for this as the midwife was very reluctant and had to go off to get the consent of the consultant on duty.

She broke my waters at 4.25pm and wanted to insert a cannula ready for the drip. I point blank refused and said she could insert it as and when I needed the drip!

She left me to it and we made the room dark with our LED candles, put on some soft music, I sat on my ball and started rotating and moving to get the contractions started. They did start within 30 minutes although after 2 hours they were still quite mild.

The midwife was really keen to put me on a drip but my view was that labour had started so there was no need. Again, I had to be quite firm and used lots of delay tactics – could we talk about it and wait an hour and then reassess?

We agreed she would give me an examination at 8pm and unfortunately, I was still only 2cm dilated. We asked for another 10 minutes to discuss the drip and by the time she came back half an hour later my body had kicked into a higher gear. 'I am a bit more convinced by your contractions', she said (I had been convinced for a while!).

But she stopped talking about the drip after that! I laboured for another hour then started using gas and air which is brilliant. There is a bit of a knack to timing it right but it took the sharp edge off the pain. I started pushing at 9.45pm and baby was born at 10.30pm.

She also had shoulder dystocia but they were ready for it and they flipped me onto my back, pushed my feet and bent my knees to open my pelvis and she popped out! I gave birth on my thick yoga mat, on the floor and didn't even LOOK at the bed!

It was the most amazing experience.

REAL EXPERIENCE: Stef's Story

I had a stretch and sweep on Tuesday morning. I went into labour on Wednesday morning, but it took until Thursday 2200 when I finally went to the hospital as I had been having 10 minute contractions since Wednesday.

I was told I was 2cm dilated and was expected back in the early hours.

I went back at 0500 on the Friday morning. I was immediately offered gas and air (which I gratefully received!)

I wanted a water birth but the pools were all in use, a temporary one was set up for me on the doctor led floor (very kindly by the staff at Royal Berks). I was in there for 4 hours by which point I was taken out to check my progress, I was still only at 5cm.

My waters were broken for me (with consent) and I went back into the pool. At this point I blacked out and the next thing I remember is being on the bed pushing (minus my gas and air). I was informed that I was only 8cm but my body had taken over, after being awake for over 48 hours I think I needed to get my boy out!

The final stage of labour took just 16 minutes, I tore (badly) and required an epidural for my stitches (as they were internal as well as external).

All in all, my labour took over 30 hours and I only used gas and air, I was told I could ask for any other pain relief at any time, and it was offered. Although I was coping so I declined.

REAL EXPERIENCE: *Emily's Story*

I started using the TENS machine when I could no longer concentrate on reading my book between contractions! It didn't exactly relieve the pain but I found it the perfect distraction, it was something I was able to focus on. Dancing to Bowie also helped!

My waters were broken artificially by the midwife as I'd been stuck at 4cm for several hours – I didn't really question it but it was a level of intervention I was happy with.

I continued to use the TENS up until entering the final stage of labour where I was encouraged by the midwife to give gas and air a try. Again, I can't be certain whether it relieved any of the pain – it was something to concentrate on.

I had been determined not to use anything 'stronger' than gas and air as I wanted to be able to remember and really experience the birth.

The thoughts which came into my head during the final stage of labour seemed more effective than any pain relief and were what really got me through, I felt connected to every woman who had ever given birth and I just knew that I could do it too. I wouldn't change anything about my first birth experience.

Chapter 17

Oxytocin Drip
(Induction and Augmentation)

What is it?

Induction of labour is where a drip with artificial oxytocin – the key birth hormone – is administered to the mother in order to artificially stimulate contractions.

The drip is administered throughout the labour until after the delivery of the placenta and the levels of the hormones can be lowered or increased to alter the effects of the drug as required.

Administering this drug to initiate and continue labour is known as *induction*. Using it once labour has begun to assist in the progression of labour is known as *augmentation*.

What happens?

A cannula is inserted into the hand or wrist and a drip is administered containing a combination of saline solution and the preferred oxytocin drug.

The two main drugs are Pitocin[126] and Syntocinon[127]. The dose can be adjusted according to the strength of contractions desired.

The mother and baby will also both have continuous foetal monitoring for the intensity of the mother's contractions and the baby's heartrate.

The use of the drugs is measured not by the maternal reaction (i.e., pain threshold) but by the heart rate of the baby. This means that the contractions can feel very strong, painful and close together from the outset, but the dose would not necessarily be reduced if the baby was not showing signs of distress.

The drug is continually administered throughout the first and second stages of labour, and the delivery of the placenta will also be managed through drugs (see Chapter 17: Active Management of the Third Stage).

When is it used?

The oxytocin drip is used if other methods of induction of labour (membrane sweep or artificial rupture of membranes) have not been successful at initiating spontaneous onset of labour.[128]

It can be used to help enhance a long or slow-progressing labour.

Induction is usually used for:

- Being over 41 weeks pregnant.
- Having certain health conditions that present a risk to the mother or baby (e.g., gestational diabetes, pre-eclampsia, choleostasis).
- Concern about the baby's growth or wellbeing.
- If your membranes have broken and labour has not started within 24 hours (to reduce risk of infection).[129]

While the use of oxytocin for inducing labour should be discussed on a case-by-case basis based on the mother's individual circumstances, it is routinely discussed with all women with non-complicated pregnancies from 38 weeks and is usually offered to all women after 41 weeks of labour. Most hospitals prefer to book a mother in for an induction by 41+4 weeks as the process can take a few days and they like to ensure all babies are born by 42 weeks' gestation.[130]

When is it not used?

The same contraindications for vaginal delivery generally would apply also to induction using an oxytocin drip:

- Vasa praevia or placenta praevia.
- Foetal malposition (e.g., breech or transverse lie).
- Cord prolapse.
- Previous vaginal rupture.
- Previous caesarean.

What are the Benefits?

The key benefit to an induction is the reduction of risks to the baby compared to if they remained in utero.

In uncomplicated pregnancies, this usually equates to the increase in risk of stillbirth (see opening section on induction) after 41 weeks.

This foetal risk can also be a result of maternal or foetal medical conditions, with a theoretical or perceived risk to the wellbeing of mother and/or baby.

It can also help a prolonged labour to progress and help to avoid caesarean section.

What are the Risks?

The risks of induction of labour using artificial oxytocin relate both to the side effects of the drugs, and also possible complications.

Drug side effects vary depending on whether Pitocin or Syntocinon are used but include[131]:

- nausea and vomiting
- headaches
- shaking
- stomach pain
- shortness of breath
- uterine rupture
- high blood pressure
- fever
- back pain
- swelling
- hyperstimulation of the uterus.

The full side effects[132] can be found on the documentation[133] for the drug.[134]

Overall effects from the levels of the drugs used can result in:

- High frequency and intensity of contractions, sometimes resulting in the contractions running together.
- Hyperstimulation of the uterus resulting in uterine rupture.
- Distress to the baby due to restriction of blood flow and oxygen.[135]

Are there any Alternatives?

There are no medical alternatives to induction other than opting for a caesarean section, and this may only be an option in certain circumstances. Many hospitals would prefer to put off a caesarean unless faced with an emergency situation.

Natural ways to increase natural oxytocin production can certainly be a good alternative to augmenting labour, however, for initiating labour itself, we can only be patient and wait for labour to start naturally.

What are the Implications?

The implications of induction are as follows.

- Hyperstimulation of the uterus can result in uterine rupture, which can be very dangerous for both baby and mother and would result in an emergency caesarean. This is extremely rare (less than 1%).

- Distress to the baby due to restriction of blood flow, which can result in either further intervention in labour or issues with the baby once born.

- General increase in risk of further intervention (30% of people induced require further assistance with either an assisted delivery or caesarean section). [136]

- Delivery of the placenta must be managed via drugs as the body's natural oxytocin delivery is interrupted.

Natural oxytocin is interrupted when you introduce an artificial version. This means that the hormones of labour are significantly affected and subsequent hormonal processes could be adversely affected. These include delivery of the placenta, lower satisfaction about the birth, bonding with the baby, breastfeeding, post-partum depression, and even a possible link to the natural oxytocin process in the body in later life.[137]

Certainly, artificial oxytocin is used for childbirth from a physiological viewpoint – to stimulate uterine contractions. However, oxytocin has a varied and complex role in the body – both physical and emotional – and the full effects of the use of artificial oxytocin are certainly not fully understood and many preliminary studies show adverse effects in many cases.[138]

It is clear that induction using artificial oxytocin is a good and necessary procedure, however it is often overused for non-medical reasons.

Inductions also often require a restriction in the movement of the mother due to the need for continuous foetal monitoring. Adopting reclined and static positions can also be detrimental to the progress of labour.

Due to the need for continuous foetal monitoring, you would also not be allowed to use water as a pain relief (i.e., taking a shower or using a bath or birth pool).

What can I do to minimise complication?

- Ensure artificial oxytocin is being offered for medical reasons or for reasons specific to the mother's circumstances rather than just routine.
- Request the minimal dose of the drug to be administered to build up the body's ability to deal with the contractions.
- Use natural methods to help stimulate the body's natural oxytocin release.
- Keep upright and mobile, allowing gravity and movement to facilitate labour.
- Try to avoid further interventions by waiting for as long as possible to use pain relief.
- Try to have plenty of tools for coping with the sensations of labour.
- Once the baby is born, try to stimulate natural oxytocin release by skin-to-skin, eye contact with baby, plentiful breastfeeding, rest, dark and warmth, with as much maternal support as possible to reduce stress.

REAL EXPERIENCE: Katy's Story

Prior to labour I was keen to avoid pain relief as far as possible and rather use breathing, movement and visualisation until I got to a point where I felt I needed something stronger.

I was induced and found the contractions after being on the drip extremely painful. After a couple of hours, I wanted to try gas and air. Unfortunately, it made me throw up and then feel extremely nauseous so I didn't continue with it. I had thought I was quite well researched but wasn't prepared for that as a side effect.

After another few hours managing with just breathing etc., I decided I wanted an epidural. Unfortunately, the anaesthetist kept being called into theatre and then changed shifts before I was able to get one.

I tried the gas and air again after that and was fine on it. I continued on it for another 5 hours before they realised the drip wasn't doing anything and I wasn't at all dilated.

At that point, we made the decision for me to have an unplanned but non-emergency c section – which they did a spinal for. It was all fine.

I can't remember the pain at all now. I stubbed my toe the morning I went into hospital and I can clearly remember what that felt like and saying to my husband, 'that's not the most painful thing that's going to happen to me today!' But for the life of me now I can't remember the pain of a contraction.

REAL EXPERIENCE: *Anna's Story*

My waters broke in the early hours of the Monday morning and contractions started a few hours later.

During the early part of labour at home I used the TENS machine, and in fact continued to use it throughout.

We went into hospital on the Tuesday morning, although labour was moving slowly so I was put on an oxytocin drip to speed things along.

Gas and air and the TENS machine worked well for me for the next few hours, but after being in hospital for 24 hours I had diamorphine which was really beneficial in my case because it meant I could get some semblance of sleep for around 4 hours.

Eventually because of the way the baby had turned I had a spinal block and ventouse and forceps delivery. The most bizarre thing was being told to push but not being able to feel what I was doing.

Although I had originally hoped to have a more natural birth I accepted that it wasn't meant to be that way for me this time, and took pain relief options based on how things were progressing.

Honestly, it's all a bit of a blur now and my hubby had to remind me of a lot of what happened. Anyway, it was all worth it to have my little boy delivered safely.

Chapter 18
Active Management
of the Third Stage

What is it?

Active management of the third stage is an injection of artificial hormones to stimulate the immediate delivery of the placenta and prevent bleeding. It is often accompanied by palpating the mother's abdomen and pulling on the cord to encourage the placenta to detach and deliver.

The injection consists of a combination of artificial oxytocin, combined with a drug called Ergometrine.[139] The brand name is Syntometrine. The effects of the drug are to stimulate a large contraction in the uterus, causing a reduction in blood flow to the uterus which has the effect of enabling the placenta to detach quickly from the wall of the uterus and helps to reduce bleeding.

As the drugs are known to pass into the baby's blood stream, immediate cord clamping is usually performed, followed by cord traction (pulling on the cord to encourage separation of the placenta).

What happens?

The injection is administered after the baby's head crowns or immediately after birth, usually into the thigh. This causes a huge contraction that makes the uterus start to shrink, cutting off blood flow and resulting in the placenta being delivered usually within 5–15 minutes.[140] (In an uninterrupted third stage, the placenta takes up to 60–90 minutes to deliver.)

Once the baby has delivered, the cord would be clamped and cut, often less than a minute after birth.

The midwife will often create traction on the cord to encourage detachment of the placenta and may massage the abdomen to encourage delivery. If bleeding continues after the placenta has delivered, a further dose of Ergometrine may be given.[141]

When is it used?

Post-partum haemorrhage (bleeding after birth) is considered by some to be one of the most dangerous parts of childbirth. While post-partum haemorrhage is very rare, it can prove to be fatal to the mother if not managed correctly.[142] It is measured in terms of mild bleeding (losing 500ml blood in 24 hours after birth) and heavy (bleeding more than 2 litres). Mild occurs in 5% of births, heavy occurs in 0.6% births.[143]

Active third stage of labour (as opposed to a physiological third stage) is known to help prevent post-partum haemorrhage and is routinely administered to women.

The injection can also be administered at any point during the third stage if bleeding occurs or if the mother has chosen to deliver the placenta more rapidly.[144]

It is always used if hormonal intervention has been used to manage the labour, or if the mother is at high risk of post-partum haemorrhage.

If a physiological (natural) third stage is chosen but the placenta has not been delivered within an hour, then often an injection is offered.

When is it not used?

Certain medical conditions are contraindicated – such as hypertension, pre-eclampsia, severe liver, kidney or heart problems. It would also not be used if you had a known allergy to the ingredients[145] or had an infection (such as sepsis).

What are the Benefits

Active management of the third stage has the following benefits.

- It reduces risk of post-partum haemorrhage, [146] although exact statistics are hard to come by due the complex combination of the active management of the third stage, combined with studies of variable quality.[147]
- It ensures quick delivery of the placenta.
- It reduces risk of anaemia.
- Many interventions earlier in labour can affect third stage and this enables the delivery of the placenta to happen smoothly after earlier interventions (such as epidural and induction with an oxytocin drip).[148]

What are the Risks?

- Side effects of the drug include: high blood pressure, nausea, vomiting, after pains (severe contractions).[149]

- Use of Synotmetrine requires immediate cord clamping as the drug passes into the baby's blood stream.

- It interferes with body's natural hormones and this can affect maternal satisfaction, plus could impact breastfeeding and bonding.

- If the cord is pulled too vigorously, it can break.

- There is also an increased risk of further vaginal bleeding in the days after birth.

Are there any Alternatives?

The main alternative is to opt for a natural third stage, known as a physiological third stage, or expectant management of the third stage.

In a physiological third stage, the cord is left to pulse, no injection is administered, and the cord is left alone. Basically, the delivery of the placenta is left to nature and the mother is left with her baby (while being closely observed).

You can also choose to have a mixed management with a combination of one or two elements of active management in combination with physiological ones. For example, you could have the injection but combine it with optimal cord clamping and no palpation.

What are the Implications?

- Mum can feel interfered with.

- The baby is not getting full benefit of optimal cord clamping and this can lead to an increased risk for a lower birth weight of baby.

- Further pain relief may be required for the after pains, as the drug can create strong contractions.

What can I do to minimise complications?

The main risks of post-partum haemorrhage seem to be associated with a longer third stage, so you can try to help this stage happen more quickly by stimulating good natural oxytocin release.

- Have immediate skin-to-skin contact with the baby.
- Have good eye contact with the baby.
- Breastfeed immediately.
- Keep warm, in a dark room with privacy.
- Adopt an upright position within 5 minutes of birth to help gravity deliver the placenta.

If you choose to have active management, or if it is part of a managed (induced) labour, you can also:

- Wait for cord to stop pulsing before having the injection.[150]
- Aid natural oxytocin release using methods outlined above.

Ensure that active management of the third stage is necessary – discuss the risks with your midwife in early labour. As active management is routinely administered in the UK, and consent is often sought at inopportune moments (as your baby is delivered), it is important to specify clearly in your birth preferences what your wishes are for this stage.

REAL EXPERIENCE: Elena's Story

For my first baby, I had an induction and epidural so I must have had the injection but can't even remember or felt it.

For my second baby, I really wanted a natural birth and I was lucky enough to have a fairly quick and easy birth with no complications. I had an idea that having the injection to deliver the placenta wasn't great but couldn't really remember why so agreed to have it.

I hardly noticed the injection itself – I had just given birth to a girl!!! – but I had really bad after pains for hours. They were so bad I needed gas and air just to cope with the pains.

I really didn't expect it would be that strong. The placenta delivered very quickly but the pain continued for 2–3 hours. Once they had subsided though, I was fine and left hospital at 3.30am, just 5 hours after giving birth!

Part 5

Assisting the Baby to be Born

The interventions and pain relief options thus far discussed are all related to aiding in the process of labour and helping the mother to cope with the sensations of labour.

In some instances, the baby needs a little bit of extra assistance at the point of delivery and so it is worth separating this into a different section.

The interventions noted in this part can be done after a completely natural labour or after any of the previous processes.

Chapter 19
Episiotomy

What is it?

An episiotomy is a cut made in the posterior edge of the perineum – the opening of the vagina towards the rear – to make more space for the baby's head to be born. It is usually made just to one side of the midline of the body (oblique), but can also be done along the mid-line as required.[151]

It can be done using a local anaesthetic, although in a situation where the baby would need to be delivered quickly, it may well be done with no anaesthetic.

What happens?

A midwife will insert two fingers into the vagina at the perineum to protect the baby's head, and then will insert a needle containing a local anaesthetic (lidocaine) into the site of the incision. Once some of the anaesthetic has been injected, she will make an incision in the perineum as required, with a pair of surgical scissors or scalpel.[152] After the delivery of the baby and placenta, the wound is sutured up using dissolvable stitches.

When is it used?

An episiotomy is used when it appears that the baby is not descending past the perineum, perhaps due to awkward positioning such as shoulder dystocia, or tilted head, to help with an assisted delivery (forceps or ventouse), as the baby is showing signs of distress and needs to be born quickly, or to avoid a natural tear.

A natural tear in the perineum is relatively common (up to 85% of births have some form of perineal trauma[153]) and can be anything from fairly minor (a graze) to severe – affecting the very deep muscles of the perineum and can tear through to the anus. This obviously causes severe pain and complications. The level of a tear is described in degrees.[154]

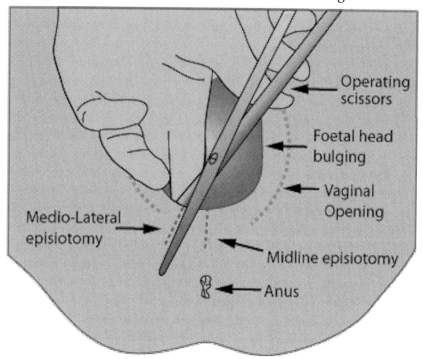

Illustration showing the two likely sites of an episiotomy.

First degree tear – involves the skin of the perineum and back of the vagina. It is quite superficial and usually does not require stitches.

Second degree tear – this tear goes a little deeper and involves the superficial muscles of the perineum. This would require stitches to repair the wound.

Third degree tear – this tear goes deeper into the perineum and partially or fully through to the anus. This would require sutures.

Fourth degree tear – the same as a third-degree tear but extends into the rectum. Extensive suturing required.

A controlled cut is thought to minimise the risk of pain and trauma to the perineum, enabling the baby to be born quickly.

An episiotomy is equivalent to a second-degree tear although the amount of tissue that is cut will depend on the individual situation. For example, if an assisted delivery is likely (forceps) then a generous cut is done to avoid a further tear originating from the cut.

It could also be indicated with a breech delivery, or if you have a medical condition that necessitated a more rapid delivery of the baby, or even after a long and exhausting labour when the mother is simply running out of energy.

When is it not used?

Episiotomies became common practice in obstetric care in the 1920s and the fashion spread rapidly with it becoming a routine procedure for most births and was as high as 52% in 1980, although has now dropped to around 15% in 2010–2011.[155]

To have an episiotomy (or not) is a difficult thing to plan for as it is usually a spontaneous act in response to a difficult delivery and is often about the opinion of the care provider and the women's choice.

There are a few contraindications to an episiotomy but they include abnormal perineum, inflammatory bowel disease, the sexually-transmitted disease LVG, and perineal scarring (perhaps due to a pervious episiotomy or tear in birth).[156]

The key contraindication is the mother's preference.

What are the Benefits?

- An episiotomy quickly makes more space so the baby can be born very quickly.
- It can help avoid other interventions, such as forceps delivery, or caesarean if that outcome looks likely.
- It may avoid a more serious tear.

It has been historically believed that an episiotomy heals better than a natural tear and also prevents more serious trauma to the perineum, incontinence and neonatal complications, although a large number of recent studies have shown evidence to the contrary. [157] [158]

Its routine use is steadily decreasing in favour of 'restricted use' i.e., used only when deemed necessary.

What are the Risks?

- It causes bleeding.

- It can tear further along the cut turning it into a third or fourth degree tear.
- It can be painful for some weeks after birth – this comprises the pain of wound, bruising, plus pain of urination/defecation.
- It has a longer recovery time than a natural tear.
- It can cause scarring that can affect sensation in the area.
- There is an increased risk of infection.
- It can cause pain or discomfort in sexual intercourse.
- It can lower pelvic floor function due to it being a cut across the muscle tissue (a natural tear usually occurs along the natural grain of the muscle and therefore heals better from a functional point of view).[159]

Are there any Alternatives?

The main alternative to an episiotomy is to avoid doing it.

There have been suggestions that applying a warm compress onto the perineum during labour can help avoid the need for episiotomy but studies have been inconclusive.

By the time an episiotomy is deemed necessary, it is usually a given that it would happen as most women put the potential safety of their baby, or avoidance of further intervention over wanting to avoid an episiotomy.

A good perspective is to avoid a prolonged second stage of labour and using techniques such as perineal massage to help avoid the need for the procedure in the first place (see section on minimising complications below).

What are the Implications?

When you have an episiotomy, it is usually accompanied with a local anaesthetic, both for the cut itself and for subsequent suturing. The administration of the anaesthetic via injection to the site can be very painful, although the suturing itself cannot be felt.

Suturing requires the mother to be in a supine position and it may not be practical for her to hold her baby during this time. Fathers or birth partners can do skin-to-skin with the baby during this time.

There may also be bruising in the area and this can make it uncomfortable or painful to sit down and walk in the days and weeks following birth.

An episiotomy requires suturing and the extent of the tear and the surgical skills of the person doing the repair can affect the level of scarring, healing and sensitivity of the area in future.

There have been incidences where suturing has not correctly lined up the tissue and this has resulted in a sensation of tugging or pulling at the scar site and sometimes future surgery to re-suture the area is required to improve comfort.

It may increase the risk of tearing along the scar in subsequent labours.

How can I minimise complications?

Prevention of the need for episiotomy

Perineal massage during pregnancy to prepare the perineal tissue for being stretched in birth can help to avoid tearing and episiotomy.[160] The aim is to soften and start to stretch the tissue in preparation of labour, much like you would train muscles for a sporting event.

Perineal massage is performed in these steps:

- Ensure thumbnails are short and hands are thoroughly clean.
- Get into a comfortable position – probably semi-reclined is best, although one leg up on a chair is also an option.
- Insert both thumbs into the vagina a few centimetres.
- Press towards the anus for 1 minute.
- Move the thumbs into a 'U' shape from the midline of the perineum and massage to the sides and back for up to 10 minutes.
- Repeat daily from 34 weeks of pregnancy.[161]

Perineal massage can be done by yourself or by a willing partner if reaching your inner vagina is difficult in the later stages of pregnancy.

There are also vaginal dilator devices (such as the 'Epi-NO'[162]) that have been developed that slowly stretch the vagina tissues through a slowly inflating balloon. Various studies[163] suggest it is another good way to prepare the tissue for labour and can help avoid episiotomy.[164]

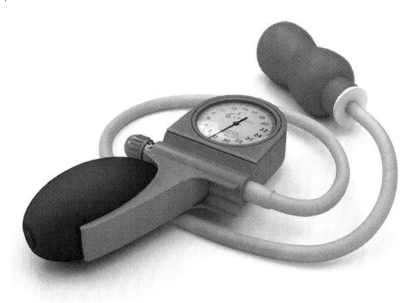

The Epi-No, a device intended to help the vagina prepare for stretching during birth.

You can also apply a warm compress to the perineum during labour in order to warm the tissues and soften them in preparation for birth. This has been shown to reduce the risk of third and fourth degree tears, although in practical terms may compromise the mother's ability to move freely and adopt upright positons during labour.[165]

Adopting upright positions during labour ensures an even pressure on the perineum during the second stage of labour and this can help reduce the need for episiotomy and/or tearing as the tissues stretch evenly[166] and gravity is able to assist in the delivery.[167] In one study the difference was 6.7% in the upright position group and 38.2% in the reclined position group.[168]

It is also helpful to avoid directed pushing – i.e., purposefully 'pushing' the baby using the whole body, rather than allowing the uterine muscles to get on with it, and following the body's natural urges to push.[169]

Minimising complications after episiotomy

The key to avoiding complications is to encourage good healing.

- Use cold compresses immediately on the area to reduce swelling and discomfort (placing sanitary pads in the fridge can be effective!).
- Use painkillers (paracetamol and ibuprofen) to reduce discomfort.
- Sit on a soft cushion or inflatable ring to keep pressure off the area.[170]

- Air the wound as much as possible.

- Ensure the wound is kept clean to avoid infection.

- Pour water over the area while urinating (avoids stinging), or hold a wet flannel on the area, or even pee in the bath or shower.[171]

- When defecating, raise the feet onto a stool to aid the body's natural position to eliminate poo.

- Start pelvic floor exercises 24 hours after birth and do them daily, even if you lack sensation in the area.

- If the wound has not healed within a month speak to your GP about the possibility of requiring antibiotics.

REAL EXPERIENCE: Kat's Story

For my first baby, I arrived in hospital 8 cm dilated (after about 6 hours of labour at home using hypnobirthing tracks).

During the examination, my waters broke with heavy meconium in it. I wanted to labour on all fours and on the floor, however the midwife was insisting on me being on my back on the bed for examinations and to monitor the baby's heart rate because of the meconium.

I started on gas and air and progressed well and was fully dilated an hour later.

Pushing was not very comfortable (on my back) and I was asked to stop gas and air, because the baby's heart rate dropped when using it.

After about 20 minutes of pushing and the baby's heart rate going up and down they did an episiotomy and the baby was there 2 pushes later.

The stitching of the episiotomy was actually more uncomfortable than the labour.

REAL EXPERIENCE: Rachel's Story

With my first baby, I was told it was best to go to the hospital when I was in agony. When I arrived after the horror stories I had heard, I was surprised to hear I was already 8cm dilated.

I only used a wheat bag, hot water bottle, a yoga ball and gas and air. I didn't feel I needed anything else. When she was ready to be born, I had an episiotomy as she was presenting shoulder first.

Chapter 20
Assisted or Instrumental Delivery

What is it?

Assisted or Instrumental delivery is assisting the delivery of the baby's head manually using either forceps or ventouse (suction cap), because the baby is in an awkward position, it needs to be delivered more quickly (second stage taking too long) or mum is too exhausted to push.

Forceps look a bit like large tongs and have beenused as a tool in childbirth for nearly 400 years.[172] Forceps are used to help to turn a baby who is not in the correct position to birth, and to help gently pull it through the birth canal.

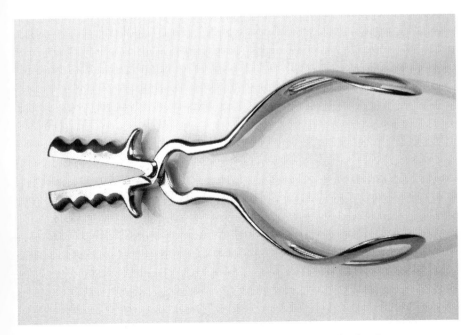

Obstetric forceps have not changed significantly for hundreds of years.

Ventouse[173] is a method of delivery that involves placing a cap upon the baby's head that is held in place through vacuum suction and is used to help extract the baby from the birth canal.

Which method is chosen will depend on the specific circumstances of the birth and the most appropriate method applied.

What happens?

The mother is placed in reclined position, with legs raised in stirrups.

The Doctor positions the forceps into the vagina and places them around each side of the baby's head in order to help reposition baby or gently pull or them.

On the case of a ventouse, a suction cap is placed on the crown of the baby's head and suction is then applied to gently pull the baby out.

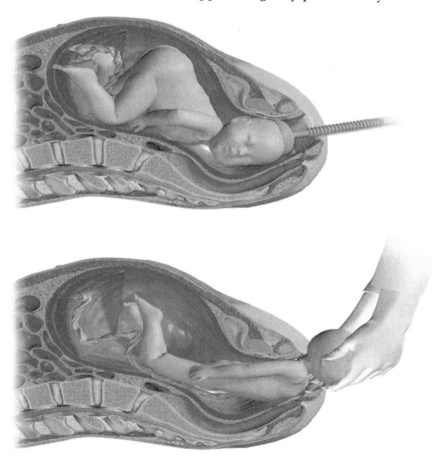

Vacuum-assisted delivery.

An episiotomy may be performed at this point to aid delivery and to avoid tearing in the perineum.

If the mother has had an epidural, it may be topped up in case of need to go to caesarean and the procedure may be performed in a surgical theatre so that if a caesarean is deemed necessary, it can be performed swiftly.

When is it used?

An assisted or instrumental delivery is usually in the second stage of labour and is performed when:

- The mother is exhausted and too tired to push during the second stage.
- The second stage is prolonged and doesn't seem to be progressing (more than 2 hours).[174] [175]
- If the mother has a medical condition that means any or prolonged pushing is dangerous.
- If an epidural has resulted in the mother being unable to push successfully.
- Maternal haemorrhage requires the baby to be delivered quickly.
- The baby is showing signs of distress and requires quick delivery.

It is only performed if the cervix is fully dilated, the membranes broken and the head fully engaged into the pelvis, and the baby was not presenting breech or brow.

When is it not used?

An assisted delivery is performed very much in the matter of opinion of the care providers. In some instances, simply a prolonged second stage is not a clear indicator of need, however a longer second stage is also associated with disadvantages for both the mother and baby.

Other contraindications include a concern about the cranial abnormalities in the foetus, or certain (rare) medical conditions of the foetus.[176]

If the baby has had internal foetal monitoring via a needle in the scalp, then ventouse would normally be avoided as the risk of bleeding from the site of the needle is increased.

What are the Benefits?

- It helps baby get into better position for delivery.
- It helps deliver baby quickly.
- Forceps is quicker than ventouse.[177]
- Ventouse does not usually require episiotomy or further pain relief.
- Ventouse is gentler on the mother and baby than forceps.
- It helps to avoid caesarean section.[178]

It is certainly clear that using an instrumental method of delivery is perceived to be a good alternative to going straight to a caesarean, although there are risks associated with both.

Overall most people would prefer to avoid a caesarean and opting to attempt an assisted delivery is preferable to major surgery.

What are the Risks?

- An episiotomy is very likely required with forceps, however probably not with ventouse.
- Perineal trauma is more likely – tearing and severe bruising, particularly if the position of the baby needs to be adjusted. In fact the position of the baby to begin with is quite relevant with regard to risk of injury.
- Further pain relief will probably be required with forceps, less so with ventouse as it is less invasive.
- It can affect continence (urinary and faecal) until bruising subsides, or longer.
- It can have a lasting (detrimental) effect on pelvic function and prolapse of the pelvic organs.[179]
- It can mark or bruise the baby's head, or cause further damage such as grazes, cuts, scarring or nerve injury. In rare cases, it can cause the eyes to misalign (strabismus, and in rare cases haemorrhage and death of the baby).
- Ventouse has a higher risk of failed delivery resulting in caesarean, partly due to the need to place the cup in a very precise location.[180]

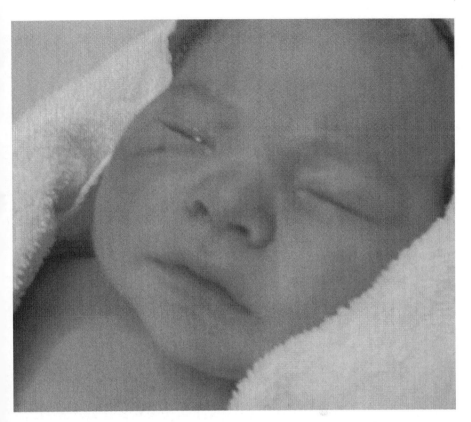

Marks from a forceps delivery.

Are there any Alternatives?

You could opt to try an episiotomy alone before including instrumental delivery and see if this helps.

Assisted delivery is not usually a course of action where there are alternatives, as a rapid delivery of the baby is considered paramount for the safety of the baby. Usually the choice of doing nothing and waiting may have an adverse effect on the baby as it is usually only considered when there is already concern.

Forceps and ventouse are alternatives to each other. The decision to use either forceps or ventouse varies depending on the need to rotate the baby's position or not (this can only be done with forceps) and the experience and preference of the care provider, although studies suggest that use of ventouse is associated with lower incidence of caesarean and perineal injury to the mother.

What are the Implications?

- Assisted deliveries generally require more and longer healing and recovery time for mother and baby than an unassisted delivery.

- The baby's head can be slightly misshapen at birth (but this goes away quickly).

- Episiotomy is likely with forceps delivery and so the complications associated with that should be considered here (see Chapter 18).

- It can affect the baby's neck and head. Some people recommend seeing a chiropractor or osteopath after birth to ensure the baby doesn't have any tight muscles.[181]

How can I minimise complications?

Remaining in an upright position and freely moving can help to avoid the need for instrumental delivery.

Avoiding opioid and epidural pain relief can also help avoid the need for assisted delivery as you are more likely to require assistance after having these drugs.

The risk is that you are 40% more likely to need an assisted delivery if you have an epidural, or if the national average for assisted delivery is 12.9%, with an epidural you have an 18.3% chance of assisted delivery.[182]

This could well be related to maternal position being reclined thus preventing mobility of the pelvis, gravity assisting delivery and generally the mother not being in a good state to push.

If you did opt for an epidural, you could try to reduce the amount of the drugs administered for the second stage, or ensure you remain in a side-lying position with open legs, perhaps supported with a ball.[183]

After an assisted delivery is performed, aftercare of the episiotomy is important and taking time to heal.

Babies can sometimes be more likely to have prolonged crying or colic after an instrumental delivery[184] as the compression of the head and stress on the cranial spine can cause discomfort or pain. This can also lead to difficulties breastfeeding.

Consulting a paediatric chiropractor or cranial osteopath can have huge benefits to the baby[185] and is worth considering in all cases of instrumental delivery.

REAL: EXPERIENCE: Briget's Story

For most of my labour, I was able to cope quite well with the pain from contractions with a combination of paracetamol and a TENS machine.

As I came into the second stage of labour, and I was assessed at home by a midwife, I requested gas and air which was great! It served its purpose and really distracted from the immediate pain of the contractions.

Unfortunately, due to the position of my baby (back-to-back), and his size, my labour stalled, and I was transferred to hospital.

When I was assessed by the obstetrician, he was fairly certain that there was enough space in my pelvis for the baby to pass through, but his positioning and my lengthy labour (resulting in my exhaustion) required some intervention, in the form of an episiotomy, and possibly a forceps delivery.

I was also asked to sign a permission to perform an emergency caesarean, but was assured that it was a 'just in case' measure. (It was –there was plenty of space for my baby to come out, he was just very awkward about doing it.)

I stayed on gas and air and the TENS machine until I was brought into theatre, when I was given a spinal block. The nurse botched the first attempt at inserting the cannula in my left hand (non-dominant), and inserted it in my right wrist instead. This resulted in a really painful bruise across the back of my hand that really interfered with my ability to stand up after I had my baby, as any pressure put on that hand hurt really badly.

After the spinal block took effect, I was numb from the waist down, and the doctors gave me an episiotomy, and because I was numb from the midriff down, needed a forceps delivery.

Fortunately, my baby was loud, large, and healthy, with no adverse effects from the forceps. Because it was 14:00 when I had my baby, I needed to stay overnight in the hospital to make sure that there were no adverse effects from the spinal block, and that I was able to pass urine on my own before I went home.

Fortunately, all effects of the spinal wore off as expected (no shakes, no after effects). Unfortunately, my baby absolutely hated being in the tiny box crib, and I was unable to sleep for the majority of my overnight stay, as he only wanted to be held. By the time I got home the next evening, I had been awake for over 48 hours, and it was a relief to hand the baby over to my husband and mother and shower and get some sleep!

An after effect of my episiotomy was that in spite of doing my best to keep the area clean and airy (which is difficult advice to follow, seeing as it's a vagina), my stitches became infected, and a few days after birth at my midwife appointment, in spite of the stitches apparently healing well on the outside, it was recommended I call my GP for a prescription of antibiotics and co-codamol for the pain I was in. This cleared any brewing infection and took care of the pain in that area.

Overall, my experience with pain relief was fairly average as far as I can tell. I was disappointed that I needed an intervention, but my husband and hospital staff were all very supportive and just wanted me to be healthy and safe, along with the baby. And in the end, we were!

I was disappointed in what ended up happening in my labour and birth. The beginnings went exactly as I had hoped (natural onset of labour, minimal pain management), but as my labour wore on, and I hit somewhere in the 34-hour range, I became too tired to cope with the pain and my resolve wore down.

I accepted the medical interventions because I was just too tired not to. Considering that I was sobbing in frustration and pain and exhaustion by the time the spinal was administered, it was probably the right call, and everyone around me was telling me that it was.

I did feel prepared for this turn of events, in a sense, but it made it no less frustrating in the end.

It's difficult to explain the sensations of labour and birth, and everyone's experience, even birth to birth is so different, and everyone's pain threshold is different as well.

People who say that they weren't really *told* about the pain of labour and birth don't really understand that it's an impossible thing to explain. It's a series of sensations so different than any other kind of pain a person will ever experience.

It's not that people are trying to keep that aspect of labour and birth a secret, it's more that they find themselves at a loss of how to explain it, because until you've been through it yourself, you can't really 100% understand.

Chapter 21
Caesarean Section

What is it?

Caesarean section is the surgical delivery of the baby from the uterus.[186] It takes around 45–60 minutes and is undertaken by an obstetric surgeon. It is usually performed using an epidural or spinal block in a surgical theatre. In this instance, the birth partner can be present at the birth. In an emergency situation, the procedure is done under a general anaesthetic and the theatre is closed to partners.

A caesarean can be undertaken before the woman is in labour, or at any point during labour if the risk to the baby or mother of vaginal birth is deemed to be too high, or the baby requires urgent medical attention.

An elective caesarean (ELCS) is planned in advance and happens before labour starts.

An emergency caesarean (EMCS) occurs at short notice during labour when there is a concern about the mother or baby that is not immediately life-threatening. In this case once a decision has been made to have the caesarean, the procedure is usually carried out within 30–75 minutes.[187] While this is known as an emergency caesarean (insofar as it is not planned), there is usually some leeway with time and the procedure is not hurried.

A true emergency caesarean – sometimes referred to as a crash caesarean – is when the baby needs to be delivered immediately due to serious concern about the wellbeing of the baby or mother. This is usually undertaken as quickly as possible after the decision to have the caesarean and in order to speed things up, a general anaesthetic is used.

What happens?

- The decision to perform a caesarean is taken and the mother is transferred to the surgical unit.

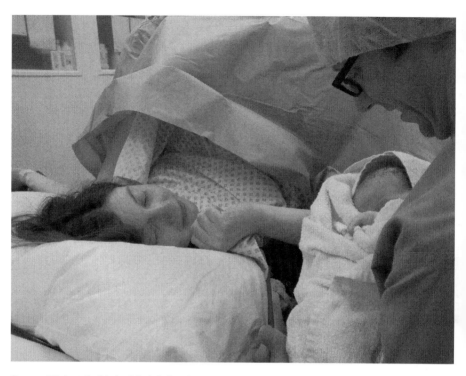

Sam and Rob at the birth of their baby via emergency caesarean.

- In an ELCS or non-immediate EMCS, the mother is taken into theatre and given spinal or epidural anaesthesia, and the birth partner is given scrubs to wear.

- In a crash caesarean, the mother is taken to theatre and given general anaesthetic (she is not conscious). In this case, the birth partner will have to wait in the waiting room.

- In all cases, the mother will have an IV drip to administer saline solution and additional drugs if required, plus a catheter inserted.

- A screen is put up at the mother's neck to block her view of the surgery.

- The mother's abdomen will be prepared for surgery with sheets to display the area to be incised and swabbed for hygiene reasons.

- An incision is made in the abdomen along the line of pubic hair (usually), through skin, abdominal muscle and uterus wall.

- Oxytocin may be administered to encourage the uterus to contract.

- The baby is pulled from the mother's belly, and in some cases forceps may need to be used. This is often in the first five minutes of the procedure.[188]

- The baby's umbilical cord will be clamped and cut.
- The baby will be assessed for wellbeing and treated accordingly if required.
- The cord will be pulled to encourage the placenta to detach from the uterus wall.
- The Surgeon stitches up the uterus wall, peritoneum, muscle fibres and skin. This can take 30–60 minutes.
- The mother will be given antibiotics to reduce the risk of infection, and steps will be taken to avoid clots (such as tight stockings for her legs and possibly anti-clotting medication).
- Once the baby is born, there is the possibility of skin-to-skin with the mother (or birth partner) and establishing breastfeeding.
- After the surgery, the mother will be transferred to the postnatal ward and will usually spend 2–3 days in hospital.

There are lots of people in the room during a caesarean section including:

- Mother
- Father
- Surgeon

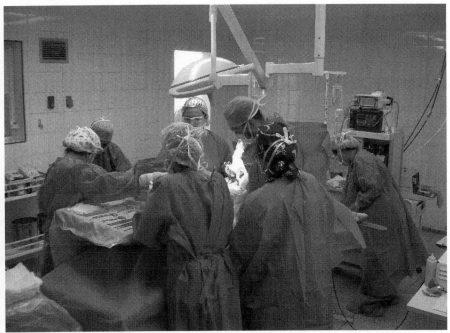

Caesarean surgical team.

- Assistant surgeon
- Anaesthetist
- Assistant anaesthetist
- Midwife for mum
- Midwife for baby
- Paediatrician
- Assistant paediatrician
- Theatre manager
- Nurse
- Students

When is it used?

An elective caesarean is used when:

- The baby is breech or transverse (although breech vaginal delivery is becoming more and more supported).
- There is a twin or multiple delivery (depends on individual circumstances).
- There are umbilical cord abnormalities.
- Placenta praevia is present, where the placenta partially or wholly covers the cervix, making vaginal delivery impossible, or other placenta issues (such as abruption or accreta).
- The mother has had a previous caesarean (although you are able to choose a vaginal birth after caesarean), or uterine rupture.
- There are certain medical conditions present (HPV virus, untreated HIV, pre-eclampsia).[189]
- Maternal request (depends on individual cases) sometimes following a previously traumatic birth, stillbirth or other risk factors.

An emergency caesarean is used when there is an immediate risk to the mother or baby in the labour. For the baby this is usually indicated by foetal distress, namely the heart rate of the baby showing concerning abnormalities (too high, too low, moving between too high or low) over a prolonged period, or very suddenly.

If the labour has been very prolonged (2–3 days) with little progress, then a caesarean may be offered due to extreme maternal exhaustion or malposition of the baby.

Other reasons include:

- If the mother has unexpected or excessive bleeding during labour.
- Cord prolapse.
- Failed induction or instrumental delivery.

When is it not used?

There is not really a list of common contraindications for a caesarean section as it is usually the best option for an ELCS and a last resort for an EMCS. In some cases where the baby is malformed or premature, then caesarean section may not be the best option, and certain cancers or infections may be contraindications.

If there is deep concern over the baby's wellbeing then it may be performed despite risks.

The biggest contraindication is the mother's choice and while in some cases it may feel that there is no choice as the risk to the baby is certain, in many cases just having a prolonged labour (for example) while being distressing and exhausting for the mother, is not necessarily an indication that a caesarean is medically necessary.

What are the Benefits?

The most obvious benefit of a caesarean section is that it delivers the baby very quickly and safely.

In the case of an ELCS, it can be a calm and beautiful experience as there is no hurry or panic and the mother completely avoids all experiences of labour, such as contraction pain, exhaustion, perineal damage. You also know exactly when your baby will be born and plan accordingly.[190]

In the case of an EMCS, labour ends quickly – as soon as the baby is born – which can be a huge relief either due to maternal exhaustion, and/or concern about the baby's wellbeing.

You can have optimal cord clamping, immediate skin-to-skin and breast-feeding in a caesarean (subject to the support of the surgical team).

You are less likely to suffer incontinence or pelvic floor issues, or vaginal discomfort during sex after a caesarean.

What are the Risks?

Caesarean section is a major abdominal surgery and there are always risks associated with such an invasive procedure. While on the one hand, it can be perceived to be a pain-free option (in comparison with labour), it nevertheless has a significant period of recovery and major implications in the postpartum period.[191]

The risks associated with epidural would also be included (unless a general anaesthetic was administered).

The list of risks with a caesarean are long, however some are uncommon.

During the procedure:

- Excessive bleeding that may require transfusion or further surgery.
- Damage to local organs (kidney, bladder, etc.).
- Accidentally cutting the baby.
- In an EMCS, if the stomach is not empty, then the risks associated with the anaesthesia are increased.
- Baby having breathing difficulties (particularly if the caesarean is performed before 39 weeks of pregnancy).
- Baby needing admission to NICU (which may well validate the decision to perform the caesarean).

After the procedure:

- Pain relief (paracetamol, ibuprofen and co-codomol) may be required.
- Deep vein thrombosis.
- The wound, or uterus can become infected.
- Internal scarring that can cause complications.
- Large abdominal scar.
- Bleeding or haemorrhage, possibly resulting in hysterectomy.
- Loss of sensation in lower abdomen or around site of scar (temporary or permanent).
- Temporary loss of bowel function, or even blockage in the bowel.
- Increased flatulence, retained gas or stool causing nausea and vomiting.

- Urinary tract infections.

- Endometriosis.

- Post-Traumatic Stress Disorder.[192]

- Increased risk of baby developing allergies, asthma[193] and obesity[194] in later life.

Future pregnancies:

- Scar stretching or opening.

- Increased risk of ectopic pregnancy.

- Increased risk of uterine rupture.

- Placenta accreta (where the placenta is abnormally attached to the uterus wall).

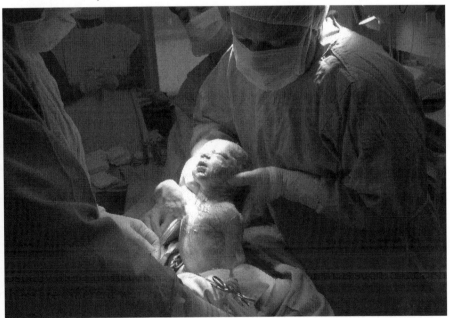

A baby is born by caesarean.

Are there any Alternatives?

Usually there are not alternatives for a caesarean birth as such, although there are different ways for them to be performed.

In all but a crash caesarean you could implement certain things to help the birth seem calmer and less clinical, and mimic a vaginal birth. This is sometimes known as a gentle caesarean.[195] Requests could include:

- Birth partner present in the room.
- Dimmed lights during the birth.
- Soft music playing or quiet voices.
- Temperature of the theatre raised (it can often be very cold in theatre).
- Talk in the theatre focussed on birth (rather than chit-chat).
- Photographing or filming of birth by partner.
- All cannulas to be inserted in one non-dominant arm, leaving the other arm free to hold the baby.
- EEC leads placed on the mother's back to leave her chest free for skin-to-skin.
- Lowering of the screen or use of a transparent screen or mirror so the mother can observe the birth.
- Baby being slowly delivered, following the uterus's natural contractions. This helps to squeeze the mucous out of the baby's mouth to help baby start breathing.
- Mother assisting in 'delivery' of baby.
- Birth partner announcing sex of baby.
- Delayed cord clamping until cord has stopped pulsating.
- Baby being placed immediately on the mother's chest (skin-to-skin).
- Breastfeeding.
- All baby assessments performed with baby on mother's chest.
- Minimal separation of mother and baby.

What are the Implications?

- You will be admitted to hospital.
- The catheter will be removed once the epidural anaesthesia wears off (12 hours after the last dose). After this you will probably stay for a further 1–3 days depending on the hospital's policy and post-operative complications.
- You are not allowed to pick up anything heavy and it can be difficult to pick up your baby in the immediate aftermath of birth, particularly when in bed.

- You are unable to drive for 6 weeks after birth.

- Scar tissue can cause pain or discomfort months or years later.

In a caesarean, particularly an ELCS, the hormonal process of labour is bypassed. This can mean that the body takes a few days to 'catch-up' hormonally. The euphoria of birth does not happen as endorphins are supressed, and the natural surge of oxytocin is affected.

This can result in late onset of lactation, difficulty establishing breast-feeding, poor bonding, and postnatal depression.

After two caesareans, you may be discouraged from attempting a vaginal birth in future. Some risks associated with caesareans also increase with each caesarean.

There has been recent research about the impact of the microbiome in newborn babies. Essentially, during a vaginal delivery, the baby collects the mother's gut bacteria through its mouth being exposed to bacteria in the mother's vagina including faecal matter present at birth.

In a caesarean, this doesn't happen and there have been studies showing that babies who have been born via caesarean have different gut microbiomes than babies delivered vaginally. It is thought that there is a link between this lack of 'seeding' of the baby's gut microbiome and increased risk of allergies and other conditions later in life.[196]

While this is a very new theory, it is being taken seriously by the scientific community and further study and research is being done.[197] There is a trend to artificially 'seed' the baby's microbiome[198] by swabbing the mother's vagina before a caesarean delivery and then placing the swab in the mouth of the baby after birth.

How can I minimise complications?

Keeping fit and active before and during pregnancy can help to reduce the likelihood of requiring a caesarean.[199]

During labour, trying to avoid induction of labour, epidural and assisted delivery can all help lower the risk of requiring a caesarean.

After the surgery, helping the body to get back on track hormonally can be done by

- Delayed cord clamping to ensure the baby gets all the blood it needs from the placenta.

- Lots of skin-to-skin[200] with the baby both immediately after delivery, and as much as possible in the first weeks, particularly while feeding.

- Breastfeeding.

- Keeping the wound clean to prevent infection.

- Chewing gum in the first 24 hours after birth to aid rapid bowel recovery.[201]

- Following advice to avoid lifting anything heavy in order to protect the wound, aid healing and prevent further abdominal muscle issues as a result of 'overdoing it'.

REAL EXPERIENCE: Celeste's Story

My labour progressed very slowly. I had contractions for about 24 hours, using a birthing pool at home which gave some good pain relief. The pain of contractions was ok, but I was getting pretty tired and it was very painful to sit or lie down so even harder to rest. I had back pain too.

I went to hospital and was only 1cm dilated so they sent me home with some codeine. I asked to be re-admitted to hospital after an hour as the codeine had no effect and more than anything else I needed some rest.

I chose to have diamorphine which dulled the pain enough that I could sleep between contractions. I had two doses that night. It was really helpful to get some sleep. Labour continued to progress very slowly so I had two diamorphine injections again the following night.

The third day I was very dehydrated and then needed a catheter. I also had back pain so didn't have any relief between contractions and was finding it hard to get into a comfortable position. I was offered water injection but felt too scared about the pain of the injection itself to go for it.

I was 11 days' overdue by this stage and had been due an induction the following day anyway if labour hadn't started. I was keen to get things progressing.

They gave me a pessary and Syntocinon injections to try and speed things up and so eventually the contractions started ramping up. I started using gas and air and had another diamorphine injection.

The gas and air was good and made me feel very distant and a bit woozy. The diamorphine let me doze a bit. I had sort of lucid dreaming – maybe a mixture of sleep deprivation, lack of food and the drugs!

However, I still wasn't progressing. My back pain was still worse than the pain of the contractions, which were like a really giant stomach cramp. It was more the lack of sleep (by now I'd been contracting for about 60 hours) that made it hard.

Eventually I decided it was worth having an epidural as if I was still not progressing I needed that relief. They wouldn't normally give it to you before 4cm dilation, otherwise I might well have had one earlier.

Unfortunately, it was a very busy night and the anaesthetist was not available so I had to wait 5 hours for the epidural. I was on gas and air all this time as we thought it best not to have more diamorphine at this point. This was the hardest section for me but I just made it through one contraction and the next and really relied on the gas and air.

Eventually I got my epidural which gave me relief and a bit of sleep. They broke my waters then to try and move things along. There was meconium in the waters.

A couple of hours in I started feeling back pain which then moved into my thigh so the epidural hadn't really worked. After trying for an hour or so to top up and move around, it still wasn't working. I couldn't feel contractions but the constant back/leg pain was quite bad.

They were going to try and re-do the epidural but by this stage I decided to have an emergency section, as I had only just made it to 4cm. Baby was doing fine, which was great, but I was pretty sure that I wouldn't have the strength reserves left to push her out even if I started progressing more quickly.

I thought it was likely I would have a C-section in the end (or at best, forceps) so I thought best to be proactive and make that decision before anything started going wrong.

The surgeon was happy with the reasons and eventually the midwife was convinced too! So instead of the new epidural, they waited until someone was available for the C-section and then gave me a spinal block for the operation.

I was scared of the epidural/spinal block process especially as you can't move and I didn't know how I could do that with the contractions! However, the yoga breathing I'd learned help me to stabilise while they were doing the injections and actually I think I didn't contract for longer time periods so I wonder whether I was somehow able to control it with the breathing.

It didn't hurt at all. The C-section was a great experience. The staff were so friendly and after the long hours of waiting suddenly it was all go and bustle.

Baby was pretty enormous which was part of the problem, though not something they'd picked up until she was born.

After the labour, I was fairly out of it and was sleeping or half asleep. But I felt fine in myself and the first few days I felt really positive, because I was so happy the labour was over!

REAL EXPERIENCE: Michaela's Story

I intended to have a home birth. I'd had a really bad hospital experience some years earlier (including lumbar puncture) and was quite hospital phobic. The midwife was quite supportive in this.

However, at 37 weeks my GP suspected that my daughter was breech. I went to the hospital for a scan to check and she was indeed a footling breech. So, I was offered an ECV the following Friday to try and turn her around.

The following Friday turned up at the hospital for them to try and convince her to turn around. She was stubborn and it failed. They had previously told us there was a risk of needing an emergency C-section during the version procedure, so we had taken everything we would need just in case.

I was then told that I would need to have a caesarean as going into normal labour would be potentially dangerous.

At this point I lost the plot completely. My husband explained why I was so distressed and after some discussion with the midwife and the consultant they decided that doing it that afternoon would be the best option for me given my emotional state. The consultant then said she could fit me in at 3 o'clock that afternoon.

In the meantime, there was a change of midwife and the one leaving briefed the new one fully on my emotional state.

So, it was 11:30 in the morning and things were set in motion. I had blood taken, medical history taken, line put in etc. The time between 11:30 and 3 o'clock flew by thankfully.

We had time to make a couple of phone calls but that was about it. My husband had to find some scrubs that fitted. Not easy, he is a big man.

At 3 o'clock I was taken down to theatre and they started operating. As it wasn't an emergency everything was done slowly and methodically. I actually started to feel relaxed surprisingly.

Everything went well. My daughter was born at 3:50. No drama, no fuss. I was sewn back up while we got to meet our little girl for the first time.

I returned to the ward and the midwives sorted me out and cleaned up my daughter.

The only pain relief I needed was paracetamol and codeine, but I think I'm unusual in that respect. I recovered very well to the extent that they allowed me to go home two days early. I was up and around and walking the following day.

Yes, it was painful but not overly so for me. I think this is because it was an elective C section not an emergency and the consultant had time to open me up and sew me back together carefully. I struggle to find my scar.

That said I don't see it as the easier option. The pain stays for quite a while. You can't drive for a few weeks after and it does restrict you.

REAL EXPERIENCE: Jenn's Story

I had two elective caesareans, both of which were conducted with a spinal block. I am diabetic and was unable to achieve good blood glucose control over my first pregnancy, which resulted in a larger than average baby.

Diabetics are much more likely to have macrosomic babies and have higher rates of shoulder dystocia. Because the estimated abdominal measurements of my baby were very large, I was advised to have a caesarean to avoid a shoulder dystocia delivery.

The situation was similar for my second pregnancy, but with the added complication of now having a caesarean scar. I agreed more readily to a C-section this time as I was also worried that my anxiety around the macrosomia would impede a natural delivery.

My experiences of spinal block and caesarean have largely been positive. Both times, the administration of the spinal block was very straightforward, quick and only caused some slight discomfort. It was fast-acting: I felt like cold water was spreading throughout my veins and then numbness up to about my chest. At some point, I was also catheterised.

With both procedures, however, I did experience a sudden drop in blood pressure from having to lie completely flat – this immediately resolved upon delivery of the baby.

I also experienced nausea – both during the operation and for 3–4 hours afterwards – but I'm not sure if that was due to the spinal block or morphine that was given (both times I was eventually given an injection to help with the vomiting).

Both procedures were very calm and there was always someone to explain what was happening or provide reassurance.

I've heard of people saying that having a caesarean felt like someone was 'doing the washing up' in their stomach, or that there was a lot of tugging. I honestly didn't feel anything...and I was surprised when they held my baby up both times because it was pretty quick! It probably took around 5 minutes from start to delivery, and then another 10–15 minutes to stitch up afterwards.

In both cases for me, my babies had a brief stay (6 hours for my eldest, 2 days for my youngest) in NICU for breathing difficulties and hypoglycaemia immediately after birth – the latter is more of an issue for babies of diabetics, but I understand breathing difficulties are quite common after C-section.

In terms of recovery, I was able to get out of bed and into a wheelchair around 12 hours after the procedure.

I was up and walking the following morning and the catheter was removed. The first time I stood up, there was a burning sensation around my scar and this persisted while walking – it got worse if I walked too far, and when coughing/sneezing/laughing.

I honestly think the best thing is to move little but as often as you can, and then build up from there – the pain subsided a little more each day, and was gone completely at 2 weeks. It's worth noting, however, that my 'core' has felt slightly weakened ever since my first C-section.

I was given strong codeine after the C-section for pain relief, but found this made both me and baby very tired.

I did persist with it for a while though as it was slightly more difficult to breast feed due to my incision being tender (lying down positions didn't work for me).

I was also given injections for 5 days afterwards in the stomach – I don't remember what the drug was, but it was to prevent blood clots.[Warfarin is administered to prevent blood clots.]

I feel quite passionately about removing the scary factor from caesareans – they can be just as calm and beautiful.

I would always be in favour of natural birth if appropriate, but I don't think any woman should feel in any way inferior for having to have a caesarean. You safely delivered your baby and that's what counts!

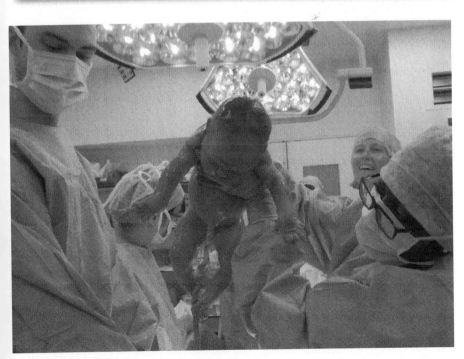

Mabel was born by emergency caesarean.

REAL EXPERIENCE: Louise's Story

I knew from the beginning of my pregnancy that I would have to have an elective Caesarean because of a neurological condition I have which prevented me from pushing.

And to be honest, this was an enormous relief from the outset, which enabled me to relax and enjoy my pregnancy more, knowing that mine and my baby's birth experience would be as stress free as possible.

A couple of times during my pregnancy I did have to shield myself from an opinion that having an elective Caesarean was some kind of 'cop out', and it would have been easy to be made to feel inadequate in some way.

Much like those mothers who either choose not to or are unable to breastfeed: If possible you just have to find a way to rise above or ignore the sanctimony.

As with most things these days, there is a lot of opinion and judgement about birth, and in some sanctimonious corners there can be found a stigma about caesarean births being lazy, or easier, but it's important to hang on to the fact that every single woman's pregnancy is different, and there are a million personal factors as to why a woman might want or need to have an elective C-section, so no one should be made to feel inadequate or lesser in some way because they are having one.

But thankfully, the number of times I encountered such opinion were minimal, and usually media based. I have to be honest and say that as my due date approached, there were a couple of times when I did feel a little bit sad at the thought of not being conscious at the birth of my child, and I was a little envious of those mothers who are able to have a C-section and remain awake, but I knew that it was much more important for us to go through the birth process as safely as possible, for both of us, and so it seemed like a very small sacrifice.

And I hope that for those mums whose labour is diverted to an emergency C-section, they can hang on to that thought, rather than feeling any disappointment, and know that they will always be the single most important being in their child's life in every other way so there really is no detriment by not being awake for that moment.

And as for the theory that those first few seconds are crucial for bonding, having a baby put to your breast immediately: codswallop and nonsense!! My son and I are as close as close can be; he was always a deeply contented, calm, happy, settled baby in every way and I absolutely do not agree with that notion one bit.

Another plus point to a general C-section is being spared all the squishing noises, the pulling and tugging and the mess!! But that is, of course, just my opinion!

For anyone who may be curious about the process of an elective Caesarean under general anaesthetic, I can only reassure you. It really is a very positive experience. You go to sleep; you wake up; your baby is there! It really is that simple! (Which is probably where all the jokes about it being a cop out come from, but hey! There are no medals for pain endurance. And you are no better or worse a parent according to the way your child entered the world.)

If anything, I choose to disregard the sanctimony as just jealousy: sour grapes!

The scar is very low down on the bikini line, and even

the lowest cut pants or trousers can't expose it. And after about a year, it is so thin and unnoticeable that you can barely see it.

The soreness of the operation is about the same duration as for a woman who has given birth 'naturally' so that aspect is equivalent to any other new mum.

For me, my son's birth by elective Caesarean was a wholly pleasant and totally stress free birthing journey and I feel very fortunate that I can say that.

Part 6
Post-birth
Interventions

Chapter 22
Immediate Cord Clamping

What is it?

Immediate or early cord clamping is when the baby's umbilical cord is clamped and cut immediately after birth.

What happens?

As soon as the baby is born, their umbilical cord is clamped with two plastic clips adjacent to another, close to the baby's body. This prevents any further blood transfer between the placenta and the baby, and minimises mess when the cord is cut. This blood transfer is known as placental transfusion.

The cord is then cut with a pair of sharp scissors (sometimes this task is offered to the father or birth partner).

The clip attached to the baby's umbilical stump remains in place until the cord stump dries up and falls off, usually within 5–15 days of birth.[202]

When is it used?

This practice first started being used in the 1930s as a way of preventing jaundice in babies, and was also hypothesised to be beneficial in preventing various other issues in newborns. These issues were subsequently disproved but with the advances in neonatal resuscitation in modern medicine, early cord clamping enabled the baby to be passed quickly to neonatal staff for treatment.

But impatience on the part of the birth physician, and a division in responsibility between the physician responsible for the pregnant mother and the paediatric one has been suggested.[203]

Ultimately, this practice became common in the UK, especially in response to using drugs to facilitate labour which can pass into the bloodstream of the baby.

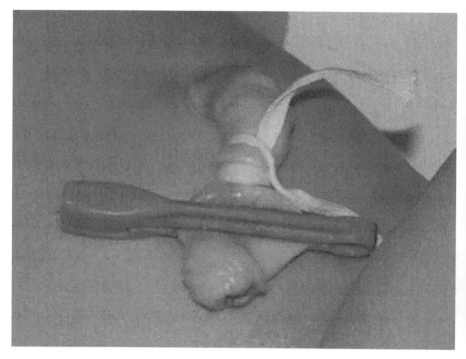

A clamped and cut umbilical cord.

In recent years, immediate cord clamping has gone out of fashion in response to overwhelming evidence showing that a delay in cutting the cord has many long-lasting benefits to the baby.

That said, there are some situations where it still may occur. If your baby's cord is compromised (ruptured or has a tight knot showing evidence that blood is not getting through), there is placenta compromise, or the integrity of the baby's heartbeat is in question (less than 60 beats per minute and not stabilising)[203], then the cord is likely to be cut quickly and the baby resuscitated by a paediatric team.

Even so, if there is any placental transfusion then it is encouraged not to be stopped as this is the baby's way of receiving oxygen.

If you have twins or your baby has certain blood conditions, then early cord clamping may be advised.

When is it not used?

Many UK and Global guidelines about immediate cord clamping have changed since 2010 in the face of plenty of evidence to show the many benefits of delaying clamping the cord. The Royal College of Midwives,[205] the National Institute of Health and Care Excellence[206], The

World Health Organization[207] and the UK Resuscitation Council[208] have all issued guidelines to encourage optimal cord clamping in nearly all situations.

Just a few years ago you had to be very specific in your birth preferences if you wanted to have optimal (or delayed) cord clamping, but most hospitals now follow these guidelines.

If you have a caesarean birth, it is still often routine to clamp the cord immediately, although if there are no contraindications, you can request optimal cord clamping. This will depend on the surgeon and so you should discuss it in advance.

It will never hurt to discuss it with your midwife and specify it on your birth preferences.

What are the Benefits?

If your baby is not receiving blood through their umbilical cord, either due to issues with the cord, or with the placenta, then cutting the cord immediately and taking the baby away to be resuscitated is an obvious benefit to get the baby's blood circulating as quickly as possible.

The same goes for if your baby's heart beat is erratic or stopped – the priority is usually to get the baby to a specialist paediatric resuscitation table.

While there are many documented studies extolling the benefits of delayed (or optimal) cord clamping, I found no studies showing any benefits to immediate cord clamping.

The only indication of benefit was in relation to bilirubin levels in the baby, which were lower in the early clamping group. High bilirubin levels are associated with jaundice in babies, although jaundice itself in the UK is not a serious concern and can be easily treated and is not considered to be a large enough risk to continue to clamp the cord immediately.[209]

In some studies there was no difference in certain factors between immediate and delayed clamping, however the clear benefits to delaying this procedure by far swing towards optimal cord clamping in most situations.[210]

What are the Risks?

The key risk with immediate cord clamping is that it prevents the baby from receiving approximately 30% of placental blood at birth. This has a variety of impacts on the baby.

- Poor circulation.

- Low blood pressure.

- Low blood volume.

- Low iron levels (anaemia) – these levels can be affected for up to 6 months.

- Low blood sugar.

- Hypothermia.

- Metabolic acidosis.

- Cardiac murmurs (rare).

- Necrotising enterocolitis (rare).

- Nearly 50% more risk of intraventricular haemorrhage.

- If the baby suffers asphyxia there is a higher risk of brain damage.

Obviously, all of these risks are mitigated to varying degrees by delaying cord clamping.

Are there any Alternatives?

Delayed, or optimal cord clamping is the alternative. The cord is left to pulsate for at least 1 minute after birth and ideally until the cord has completely stopped pulsating – usually within 10–15 minutes, and then it is clamped and cut.

The consensus in the UK now is that this 'alternative' option is becoming the norm. It would never hurt to be clear to your birthing team in your birth preferences if you would like to make sure optimal cord clamping is undertaken.

What are the Implications?

The main implications of immediate cord clamping are:

- The baby's blood (and therefore oxygen) supply is cut off immediately. If this is before the baby has started breathing on its own, it could compromise their oxygen levels and they may require resuscitation.

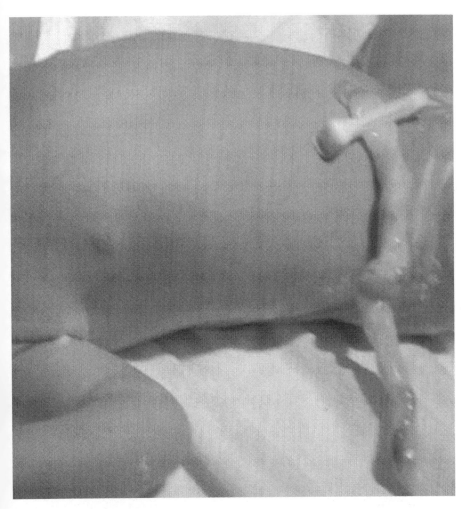

A clamped umbilical cord that has been left to pulsate for 3 minutes

- The baby has around 30% less blood than when the cord is left to pulsate. This can have an effect on the baby's iron levels for up to 6 months.

- The baby is no longer 'connected' to the mother through the umbilical cord and so can be taken away from the mother, for example, to be examined or weighed.

How can I minimise complications?

If you opt for immediate cord clamping, you can do the following to ensure that complications are minimal:

- Request that the baby is kept close to the mother, preferably with skin-to-skin contact.

- If the baby needs resuscitation, request that they are brought back to the mother as soon as possible for skin-to-skin contact.

- If the mother needs medical attention, request that the father/birth partner can have skin-to-skin with the baby as soon as possible.

- If there is any concern about the iron levels of the baby, take advice from your GP or health visitor. Breast-fed babies, and babies fed with formula milk will absorb enough iron to keep their iron levels sufficient. [211]

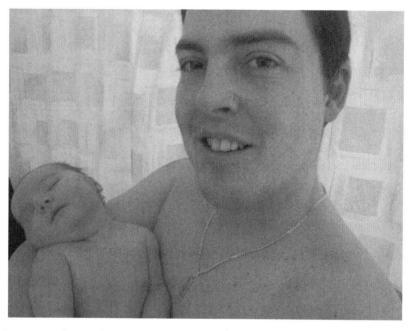

Fathers can have skin-to-skin with the baby if the mother needs medical attention.

REAL EXPERIENCE: Faye's Story

I had a sweep on Monday, then again on Wednesday which brought me to 1cm dilated. My waters broke on Thursday evening. I called the delivery unit at RBH and was advised that if contractions hadn't progressed significantly in 24 hours I should call again to be admitted as broken waters could lead to infection.

What I didn't realise at the time is that they were PROM waters (pre-waters behind the baby's head). Therefore, my actual waters were yet to break during the delivery.

I was admitted on Friday evening. Only just though as they were shut due to staffing on over admittance. Nearly went to Swindon!!! Not great for the stress levels!!

Once I was admitted to RBH the midwife attempted to examine my cervix. However, I have a very high lying cervix and she couldn't find it.

It took several rather painful attempts to find it. She kept trying to pull it down. OMG the pain! Yes, my cervix is attached to my uterus! Pulling and tugging it down is really quite painful!!!

Finally, she gave up and put the pessary in to start the contractions i.e. begin the induction process. It took a while to get started but the pessary got the contractions working and I was admitted to the delivery ward.

I spent the entire night on my own in a bed with a TENS machine in agony!! At 6am the nurse came to check on me as I was whimpering like a child!

She examined me. Where is your cervix??? Prod, pull poke, ouuuuuchhh!!!!! OK you're 4cm dilated, you're officially in labour, down to the delivery suite for you!

I had a combination of the TENS machine and gas and air. The gas and air was great and helped with the pain relief.

I was able to move around and bounce on a ball for most of the morning. But the midwife wanted to monitor me more closely so asked me to get on the bed.

The contractions towards the end, i.e., between 8-10cm, weren't progressing fast enough so she put me on a drip to speed up the process.

In the meantime, the baby's heart was dropping so I had to get up in the stirrups, had the episiotomy, and forceps to get the baby's head out as the cord was wrapped around her neck.

Immediate cutting of the cord as it was around her neck. Injection in the bum to deliver the placenta. Done...oh and 30 mins of stitches double OUCH! But I finally got to hold my Audrey.

Chapter 23
Vitamin K

What is it?

Vitamin K aids in blood clotting. Adults get it from eating dark green leafy vegetables (90%) and the rest naturally occurs from our gut bacteria.

Babies are known to have very low levels of vitamin K at birth, and as breastmilk also has very low vitamin K levels there is a risk that the baby may have a vitamin K deficiency. This deficiency can have serious complications, namely a condition known as Vitamin K Deficiency Bleeding (VKDB).

VKDB can have very serious complications –uncontrolled bleeding in the brain – that can lead to brain damage and even death. However, VKBD it is very rare and it is difficult to identify clear risk factors. It can happen in the first 8 weeks of a baby's life and is classified into early (within 24 hours), classic (1–7 days), or late (1–8 weeks) onset.

The risk of VKBD varies across these three classifications. Early VKBD seems to be exclusively found in babies whose mothers have been taking drugs that inhibit vitamin K production and/or absorption.[212]

Classic VKBD is usually associated with problems with feeding. It is very rare and occurs in only 0–0.44% of babies who have not received any vitamin K.

Late VKBD is the most serious but still incredibly rare with a rate of only up to 10.5 infants out of 100,000 (that is just) 0.0105% of cases.

Nevertheless, despite being incredibly rare it is a very serious condition. Therefore, babies in the UK are recommended to have a vitamin K dose at birth as a preventative measure to avoid any possibility of vitamin K deficiency, and VKBD.

While parents do have to provide consent, most do without being fully informed on what vitamin K injections do.

What happens?

Vitamin K is administered most commonly through an injection in the top of the thigh in the first few hours after birth – usually within 24 hours.[213] This is administered by the midwife attending the birth. This method is the most efficient method of administering vitamin K.[214]

It can also be administered through an oral dosage. A small glass vial containing the dose is opened, and poured into the back of the baby's mouth/throat.

This method is processed more quickly by the body and so three doses are usually given on days 1, 7 and 30 but can slightly vary. The initial dose is given by the birthing team and then the parents need to visit their GP to get a prescription for the other two doses, and they self-administer them at appropriate intervals.[215]

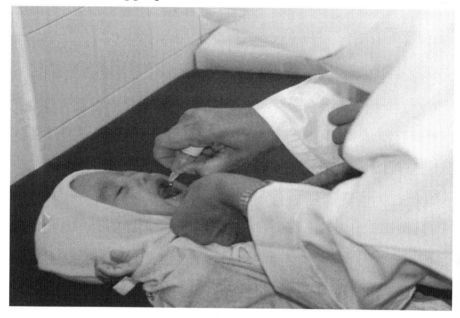

Oral Vitamin K is administered.

When is it used?

Risk factors for vitamin K deficiency are[216]:

- Maternal medicines that interfere with vitamin K production.
- Premature babies (born before 37 weeks).
- Instrumental delivery (forceps, ventouse or caesarean) that could

cause bruising.

- Babies who were deprived of oxygen at birth.

- Suboptimal breastfeeding.

An injection is routinely administered at birth unless the parents specifically request an oral dose. Parents can refuse a vitamin K dose altogether.

When is it not used?

There are very few instances where it would not be used, essentially if there was a known allergy to vitamin K itself or any ingredients in the injection (unlikely), or if the parents wished to opt out of the injection.

What are the Benefits?

Clearly the key and only benefit is that it virtually eliminates the risk of VKBD. While it is impossible to predict which babies will develop VKBD, it is 100% treatable and preventable through this dose.

The benefits of the injection are that it is a one-time shot that is administered at birth and then you can forget about it. It releases vitamin K slowly and will be sufficient for the baby until they are mature enough to acquire it through food.

The benefits of the oral dose are that you avoid giving your baby an injection at birth.

What are the Risks?

The risks of the injection appear to be nil. Some parents feel uncomfortable about the other ingredients of the injection but generally they are either natural ingredients or approved as safe. If you are concerned about the ingredients then you should ask your midwife or GP for the brand name of the injection used so you can research the specific ingredients.

I could find no information regarding side effects of the injection because they are either non-existent or extremely rare (and possibly related to another condition or illness).

Therefore, the risks I am going to comment on are associated with choosing an injection versus an oral dose of vitamin K.

The risk of the injection is that it may cause your baby pain and discomfort, and may give the baby a mild bleed or bruise at the site of the injection.

The risks of the oral dose are that you the have to obtain a prescription for the second two doses from your GP (meaning a trip to the GP before day 7), administering the dose yourself, and remembering to administer both doses at the appropriate time. The baby could spit or vomit up the dose, thus decreasing its efficacy.

Are there any Alternatives?

The only alternatives are not having the vitamin K dose at all, or choosing between an injection and an oral dose.

How can I minimise complications?

If you choose the injection, you can breastfeed the baby during the injection to help comfort them. You can also press firmly on the injection site to prevent bleeding or bruising.

If you opt for the oral dose, you can ask if the midwife or GP would be happy to give you a prescription immediately to save a GP visit. You could also ask if the GP would be happy to administer the dose, although most will prefer the parents to take responsibility.

REAL EXPERIENCE: Bea's story

I had a straight-forward natural birth but hated the idea of my baby being given an injection immediately so we opted to have the oral dose of Vitamin K.

The first dose was given by the midwife on the day after she was born at our home visit. Then we had to make an appointment with our GP to get the prescription for the second and third doses. We had to go straight-away as the second dose is due after a week but getting an appointment at our surgery is pretty difficult!

We got to the GP and they were a bit baffled by the whole thing – apparently, it is very unusual to opt for an oral dose of vitamin K. I can see why as it is a bit of a faff!

They had to look up what to prescribe and we were a bit surprised when they told us we had to give the baby the dose rather than being done by a nurse.

The prescription was two glass vials. You had to crack off the top and just pour it in her mouth. In the end, it was very easy.

I could see that if you had a difficult birth or caesarean section, it would be very difficult to pick up the prescription and next time I think I would just opt for the injection to be honest as it is so much easier and you can just forget about it.

Part 7
Postnatal Healing

As the statistics show, over half of us will choose some form of intervention in birth, from a few puffs of gas and air right through to an induction, epidural and caesarean section.

In some cases there will be choice and in some the decision will be made from concern about the welfare of the baby or mother.

Physical healing

Even with a completely natural birth, the body can undergo injury such as minor or major tearing of the perineum (the flesh around the vagina and anus), grazing, bruising and exhaustion. In most cases these are small problems that don't require further treatment but can involve a few stitches.

In general birth wear and tear, the best way to promote rapid healing is to:

* rest as much as possible,
* cold compress on the vaginal area,
* lavender essential oil applied.

In cases where bigger interventions have occured, the risks of injury are somewhat bigger due to the nature of the intervention (for example, episiotomy), or the way a more hands-on approach is taken to assist the baby (as in forceps delivery).

In these cases, the delicate tissue around the vagina, vulva, perineum and anus can be bruised, grazed, torn or cut, or a mixture of them all. There may also be sites where a cannula has been inserted (induction or epidural), and with a caesarean section, major abdominal surgery has been performed.

It is crucial to follow the healing advice of your medical team - particularly for a caesarean - but here are some additional ways in which you can encourage physical healing.

- Rest , rest, rest - not just sleep but avoiding housework, especially strenuous work like vacuuming or changing the beds. You will lose sleep with a newborn baby anyway, so right from the start your body is in rest deficit. Do as little as possible for as long as possible.

- Take warm baths with lavender essential oils (once cleared by your medical team if you have had a caesarean).

- Eat good healing foods with plenty of vitamins and minerals - fresh fruit, vegetables and home-cooked food.

- Be the boss of your visitors - put them to work. They can make you a cup of tea, and would they mind just doing a bit of washing up while they are there.

- Sit on soft cushions, or even a blow up ring to keep pressure off your vulva.

- Prop your feet on a low stool while going for a poo - this helps to get the body in the best position to release, and eating prunes and fruit to keep your poo soft is also a great idea in the early days!

Be on the lookout for poor physical healing. Most bruising, tears and stitches should settle down within a few days, caesarean scars obviously take much longer to heal, but should show signs of healing quickly.

If within a few weeks you are still in discomfort of perineal injury, get checked out by your GP.

If you notice any new or increased redness, swelling, soreness, lumps or pus, or you start to show signs of fever, then contact your midwife immediately. Most infections can easily be treated with a short course of antibiotics.

It is very hard to adapt to motherhood, and deal with emotions around birth, when your body is not healing properly.

Emotional healing

In my opinion, apart from real genuine emergencies which can be terrifying, especially if it has been difficult for you to conceive, one of the key drivers of emotional trauma is having a birth that didn't go to plan.

To have chosen interventions when your intention was to be natural; to have not been able to cope with the sensations of labour; to feel out of control and unsupported in the labour room.

Postnatal trauma can take many forms - there is a book here in itself - but it is absolutely normal to feel negative emotions about your birth.

Many women find they experience feelings of failure for not being able to cope with the pain, of not sticking to their principles, and that their body had failed in giving birth, unlike millions of women before them who managed a natural birth.

This is a completely understandable mindset and many people will dismiss those emotions - either in someone else, or more commonly in themselves - by expressing gratitude that their baby was born safely above all else, and that their reaction of guilt or failure is something to hide.

In fact, the safe arrival of a baby is a given to me - no-one on earth wants their baby to be in any kind of danger, however, it is entirely valid to feel a variety of emotions about your own birth experience. Milli Hill, the founder of the Positive Birth Movement, has written a brilliant article that discusses this in far better words than I can manage. Google, 'A healthy baby is not ALL that matters'.

It is OK to feel: guilt, a sense of failure, disappointment, remorse, regret and even grief. Hiding these feelings is not healthy and being open to family and friends about your feelings and seeking support will do wonders for your mental health.

Having a newborn baby is a wonderful but also stressful time as you adapt to a completely new life that no-one can prepare you for. Having emotional trauma to deal with as well can make the experience of new motherhood far from enjoyable.

For some women, they are so traumatised by their birth experience that they find it impossible to talk or even think about it without being overwhelmed and get very upset.

For some these feelings fade as motherhood kicks in, but for others thay can linger and intensify. Seeking help from family, friends, breastfeeding supporters, midwives, health visitors and doctors is the best step you can take.

Strong negative emotions can tip over into more serious mental illness such as post-traumatic stress disorder, postnatal depression and post-partum psychosis in severe cases. Medical help is strongly advised if you suspect you may be suffering from any of these issues, or that your emotions are greater than you can cope with.

Symptoms of depression and postnatal ill health to look out for are[217]:

- Emotional

- Low mood for a long period of time
- Irritability
- Lack of interest in your new baby and/or yourself
- Feeling alone
- Feeling useless, worthless and guilty
- Feeling overwhelmed with situations

Mental ability

- Panic attacks
- Lack of concentration and motivation
- Flashbacks

Physical

- Difficulty sleeping or feeling constantly tired
- Tension – headaches, stomach pains or blurred vision
- Decrease in appetite or increased appetite
- Reduced sex drive

If you suspect that you may be suffering from postnatal anxiety, depression, or psychosis, the best thing to do is seek immediate help. Call your midwife, health visitor or GP and demand an immediate appointment.

Alternatively, there are helplines available to advise and support you such as the MIND helpline 0300 123 3393 (UK). (Obviously organisations and phone numbers will vary in countries outside the UK. Just google 'postnatal depression with your country name and you should find plenty of places to seek support.)

Another fantastic option after a difficult birth is to ask for a birth review from your local hospital. This can be done at any time after a birth - even years later.

You can request to get a copy of all your notes from the birth - many hospital trusts will charge an administration fee for this - and you can also request that a midwife talks through the notes with you to help you make sense of what happened.

Even though your memories may feel very vivid, it is surprising how having a professional and objective view of what happened from a medical point of view can help you to understand the sequence of events, perhaps why interventions were needed (this is often not very clear in the throes of contractions), and can help to show you that you made the best decisions and choices at the time.

If you want to access your notes a good place to start is to contact your hospital's Patient Advice and Liason Service (PALS) who will be able to point you in the right direction. You can either access your notes and take them to an independent midwife or doula to talk through them with you, or request a debrief with someone from the hospital.

Most hospitals will have information about this somewhere on their website.

Looking ahead to motherhood

A key part of postnatal healing is to facilitate your ability to make peace with your experience and to be able to look ahead to motherhood, rather than be stuck looking back at the birth.

Joining mum and baby groups like postnatal yoga, music, sensory, and even just hanging out at the park gives you a great opportunity to meet other mums who are most likely going through the same physical and emotional healing as you.

Social media can also play a part in this and I have found belonging to a Facebook Group of mums an invaluable place for advice and support, venting and having fun.

Through my business, Birthzang, I have created a very successful and supportive community called 'Birthzang Mums' Club', which is open to any mum, in any location, who would like to be a part of a network of non-judgemental mums. Feel free to join at www.facebook.com/groups/birthzangmumsclub.

Seeking support in any way can only give good outcomes and if you are shy to make friends then an online forum is a great way to start.

REAL EXPERIENCE: Briget's Story

In my first birth I had an episiotomy. It was unexpected and I had a very long labour with a handful of complications, and by the time they wheeled me into theatre I was exhausted and frustrated by the way my son was about to be born, but had given in to the fact that he needed a little help getting into the world.

Unfortunately, my episiotomy ended up becoming infected, which became apparent somewhere around day 3 postpartum, and was confirmed by the midwife at my appointment in the postnatal clinic when she looked at my stitches.

There were no obvious signs of infection, but the stitches were swollen and tight, and my pain indicated that something wasn't healing quite right below the surface. At that point, sitting and standing were extremely painful for me.

The midwife recommended that I call the GP and have antibiotics prescribed for the brewing infection, and co-codamol for the pain. After that, the stitches seemed to heal brilliantly.

It was frustrating that this was just one more thing that made my first son's birth not the happy and triumphant thing I had been hoping for.

It felt like my body had failed me in almost every way bringing this beautiful boy into the world, and it's taken me a long time to accept that.

In my second birth, I managed to have a natural birth using gas and air and paracetemol as my only pain management during the actual birth, and ended up with a second degree tear. The midwife who stitched me up was quick and efficient and talked me through what she was doing. It hurt to have the anaesthetic administered, but then the stitches were just the weird plucking sensation.

The stitches from my tear healed much better than the stitches from my episiotomy. There was never any sign of infection, and no particular discomfort other than the general discomfort of having passed an 8 lb 14 oz melon through an opening the size of a baseball.

I think I was definitely traumatized a little bit by my first labour and birth. It's easy for me to tell the full story out loud, but it's still difficult for me to put it into written words.

REAL EXPERIENCE: Katy's Story

I had two very different c section recoveries.

First time round I had had a non emergency but unplanned c section following a failed induction. I had been on a drip for 12 hours before the section and hadn't slept in a couple of days.

Recovery was really hard. I had problems feeding, the baby lost 'too much weight' and we kept being borderline for various things which all meant I had to go to the hospital or gp 2-3 times a week for the first few weeks.

Walking to all the appointments, getting the pram in and out of the doctors with no step free access meant my scar took weeks to heal.

No one has a proper overview of you postnatally so each department asking us just to pop back 'just in case' one *more time was unaware of the impact on me. And I was too knackered to argue.*

I ended up with a seroma (build up of fluid) behind the scar which got infected, causing the scar to burst rather dramatically in the middle of the night.

Cue more appointments and trekking to and from the drs/ hospital.

We don't have family living locally and it was a really difficult isolating time. It took over 2 months for me to begin to feel normal and be able to get out and build a support network.

Second time around we were told there was only a 50% chance of delivering naturally.

While I didn't want another section after what had happened before, on reflection I thought it was best to have an elective section than risk a long labour followed by an emergency.

But we needed a strategy to avoid such a horrendous recovery - especially with a 2 year old at home.

I was relatively well rested going into surgery. My husband and I had agreed a strategy for avoiding any unnecessary appointments after the birth - being more challenging with health professionals without jeopardising anyone's safety.

I listened to my body far more and was better at reading when I was about to overdo it. As a result, recovery has been so much easier - both mentally and physically.

I have been able to enjoy the first few weeks far more than I did the first time round.

Part 8
Preparation and Education

My aim in writing this book is not to encourage women to choose pain relief and interventions, but rather to provide full and impartial information about what those choices involve.

Some, as we have seen, have very little impact on the mum and baby and can be a fantastic way to cope with labour. Others have much more widespread implications and risk.

What has driven me to write this book is the way that these weighty decisions to choose pain relief - such as epidural, or to have interventions such as an induction of labour - are often made with very little prior knowledge of what is involved. We make huge decisions around our bodies in labour and birth with little or no idea of the consequences of those decisions.

Our doctors and midwives don't have enough time to carefully explain the pros and cons of every decision and rely on us to educate ourselves. And while much of that information is freely available on the internet, getting a really in-depth, impartial summary is quite hard.

One of the greatest barriers to a positive birth is fear, and fear is driven by ignorance. Once you educate yourself with knowledge about birth itself, and all the ways we can give it a helping hand, and how those ways can affect birth, we immediately take away the fear.

If we understand fully what an induction of labour is, what all the stages consist of, how long it could take and what the benefits and risks involved are, then we can begin to make really good decisions about what is best for our baby and our body.

We can stop taking a doctor's word for it, and take back control in the labour room by really understanding everything that is said to us and knowing when it is being offered out of policy or need.

We can empower ourselves - and our birth partners - to stay calm during labour, to do all we can to enhance the natural process, and also to decide what pain relief and interventions are going to work best for us based on our own personal situation.

We can begin to respect and appreciate the body's natural processes and understand when we just need to be patient, or try something else, or if something is actually going wrong.

If we make informed choices and decisions about using pain relief in labour and intervening in the natural labour and birth processes, then we help to reduce trauma and anxiety around childbirth as a result of feeling a loss of control.

Knowledge eliminates fear and gives us power.

I hope this book goes some way to educate you, empower you, give you tools to make the best decisions for your labour and birth, and enter motherhood with a positive and self-assured mindset.

There is no failure only feedback

I want to make sure that this book has achieved all that I hope it to, but the only way I can find out is by getting your feedback.

If you have any questions or concerns about any topic covered in this book then I am more than happy to personally answer questions, or signpost you to relevant resources.

You can email me at eleanor@birthzang.co.uk and I will respond to every message.

Please note I am not a medical professional and cannot offer medical advice. I am, however, trained as an Active Birth antenatal teacher, have 2 children and personal experience of pain relief and birth interventions, and have worked with over 600 mothers from pregnancy into motherhood. I can help you to educate yourself as best you can to make the right choices for you.

I have written numerous blog posts on a variety of topics relevant to pregnancy, birth, and parenthood. Pop over to www.birthzang.co.uk/blog and check out some of my most popular blogs, such as 'using Clary Sage Oil in Labour', and 'Birthzang's Amazing Baby Fart Expulsion Technique'.

If you have enjoyed this book, please leave me a review on Amazon. It helps others to understand if this book is going to help them educate themselves and make the right choices in their labour and birth.

Useful Websites for Further Research

Association for Improvements in the Maternity Services (AIMS)

www.aims.org.uk

A website providing information and support about maternity choices, raising awareness of relvant issues and protecting women's rights in childbirth.

Birth Choice UK

www.birthchoiceuk.com/Professionals

This website has all hospital statistics across the UK around labour and birth.

Birth Rights

www.birthrights.org.uk

An organisation dedicated to improving women's experience of pregnancy and childbirth by promoting respect for human rights.

Cochrane Library

www.cochranelibrary.com

A collection of six databases compiling high-quality independent evidence to inform healthcare decision-making.

Evidence Based Birth

www.aims.org.uk

Association for Improvements in the Maternity Services (AIMS)

AIMS has many leaflets about all aspects of labour and birth.

National Childbirth Trust (NCT)

www.nct.org.uk

This is a UK-based charity providing information on pregnancy, child birth, breastfeeding, and parenthood.

National Institute for Health and Care Excellence (NICE

www.nice.org.uk

NICE provides national guidelines for hospitals on all medical proce dures. It includes many further references to research.

National Center for Biotechnology Information (NCBI)

www.ncbi.nlm.nih.gov

A huge database of studies with access to millions of journal articles and research papers.

NHS Choices

www.nhs.uk/pages/home.aspx

This website provides information on all medical conditions and procedures.

PANDAS Foundation

www.pandasfoundation.org.uk

A support service for families suffering prenatal/antenatal and postnatal illnesses.

The Positive Birth Movement

www.positivebirthmovement.org

An organisation that aims to promote the idea of a positive birth for any woman in any birth circumstance through recognition that appropriate support and respect is the best way to ensure a positive birth experience.

Royal College of Midwives (RCM)

www.rcm.org.uk

A wide range of research articles of current procedures and practice and other relevant research.

Image Credits

Chapter 1
A birth scene from 1800. Credit: Unknown Wellcome Collection.

Most babies in the UK are born in a hospital or midwife-led unit. Credit: Pixabay.

Chapter 2
Midwives have an uncanny ability to quickly build up a rapport with parents. Credit :Salim Fadhley, https://www.flickr.com/photos/salimfadhley/.

Chapter 4
The cervix opening in the first stage of labour. Credit: By OpenStax College [CC BY 3.0 (http://creativecommons.org/licenses/by/3.0)], via Wikimedia Commons.

Opioid-based drugs can help to relieve pain. Credit: Kala Bernier, https://www.flickr.com/photos/thisstupidlamb/.

The baby is expelled from the body during the second stage. Credit: OpenStax College – Anatomy and Physiology, Connexions Web site.http://cnx.org/content/col11496/1.6/, Jun 19, 2013.

The placenta is delivered once the baby is born. Credit: OpenStax College – Anatomy and Physiology, Connexions Web site.http://cnx.org/content/col11496/1.6/, Jun 19, 2013.

Chapter 5
An Elle TENS machine, designed to be used in labour. Credit: Eleanor Hayes

Showing the appropriate placement of TENS pads on the back. Credit: Eleanor Hayes

Siobhan found the TENS machine useful in early labour and used it while distracting herself with a large jigsaw! Credit: Siobhan Marsh.

Chapter 6
A cylinder of Entonox with a demand valve nozzle (bottom of image). Credit : By Owain Davies (Own work) [CC BY 3.0 (http://creativecommons.org/licenses/by/3.0)], via Wikimedia Commons.

Credit: Anna Hutt.

Chapter 7
Intradermal injection. Credit: By Medical Marketing Berlin GmbH (Medical Marketing Berlin GmbH) [CC0], via Wikimedia Commons.

Chapter 9
An epidural administered in the lumbar region of the back into the epidural space. Credit: By BruceBlaus (Own work) [CC BY-SA 4.0 (http://creativecommons.org/licenses/by-sa/4.0)], via Wikimedia Commons.

An epidural is administered by an anaesthetist. Credit: MrArifnajafov [GFDL (http://www.gnu.org/copyleft/fdl.html) or CC BY 3.0 (http://creativecommons.org/licenses/by/3.0)], via Wikimedia Commons

Jyoti found great relief after having an epidural. Credit: Jyoti Shule.

An epidural can help you get some much-needed rest. Credit: Eleanor Hayes.

Charlotte lay on her side with her upper body propped up during her epidural to try to keep her pelvis mobile and allow gravity to help her baby move down. Credit: Charlotte King

Chapter 10
A midwife checks the baby's heartrate at a home birth. Credit: By Pumpkingood (Own work) [CC BY-SA 3.0 (http://creativecommons.org/licenses/by-sa/3.0)], via Wikimedia Commons.

A typical CTG output for a woman not in labour. A: Fetal heartbeat; B: Indicator showing movements felt by mother (caused by pressing a button); C: Fetal movement; D: Uterine contractions. Credit: By -- PhantomSteve/talk | contribs\ (The original uploader was Phantomsteve at English Wikipedia) - I (-- PhantomSteve/talk | contribs\) created this work entirely by myself. (), CC BY-SA 3.0, https://commons.wikimedia.org/w/index.php?curid=19780765.

Delyth had foetal monitoring to check the heartrate of her baby. One monitor is for the baby's heartbeat, the other for the mother's. Credit: Delyth Mair Edwards.

Siobhan was monitored and also had a cannula inserted in case she required the use of remfentinol as she was contraindicated for pethidine or epidural. Credit: Siobhan Marsh.

Staying upright is possible with continuous monitoring. Credit: Nick and Dana Blizzard, https://www.flickr.com/photos/blizzardfx/.

Chapter 11

A vaginal examination (outside of pregnancy). Fingers are inserted and the cervix is assessed through judging how far apart the fingers can go which is very subjective. This image shows a non-pregnant body. Credit: By Unknown photographer/artist (National Cancer Institute, AV Number: AV-0000-4114) [Public domain], via Wikimedia Commons.

Chapter 18

Illustration showing the two likely sites of an episiotomy. Credit: The original uploader was Jeremykemp at English Wikipedia - Transferred from en.wikipedia to Commons by Jalo., Public Domain, https://commons.wikimedia.org/w/index.php?curid=3751824.

The Epi-No, a device intended to help the vagina prepare for stretching during birth. Credit: Epi-No https://epi-no.co.uk/

Chapter 19

Obstetric forceps have not changed significantly for hundreds of years. Credit: http://wellcomeimages.org/indexplus/obf_images/b1/b0/802abe8ee06f438c50e969fd8e25.jpgGallery: http://wellcomeimages.org/indexplus/image/L0058090.html, CC BY 4.0, https://commons.wikimedia.org/w/index.php?curid=36207542.

Vacuum-assisted delivery. Credit: By BruceBlaus (Own work) [CC BY-SA 4.0 (http://creativecommons.org/licenses/by-sa/4.0/)], via Wikimedia Commons.

Marks from a forceps delivery. Credit: Eleanor Hayes.

Chapter 20

Sam and Rob at the birth of their baby via emergency caesarean. Credit: Sam Wade and Rob White.

Caesarean surgical team. Credit: By Bobjgalindo (Own work) [GFDL (http://www.gnu.org/copyleft/fdl.html) or CC BY-SA 4.0-3.0-2.5-2.0-1.0 (http://creativecommons.org/licenses/by-sa/4.0-3.0-2.5-2.0-1.0)], via Wikimedia Commons.

Mabel is born by Caesarean Section. Credit: Sarah Sheen

A baby is born via caesarean section. Credit: By Astaffolani (Own work) [GFDL (http://www.gnu.org/copyleft/fdl.html) or CC BY-SA 4.0-3.0-2.5-2.0-1.0 (http://creativecommons.org/licenses/by-sa/4.0-3.0-2.5-2.0-1.0)], via Wikimedia Commons.

Chapter 21

A clamped and cut umbilical cord. Credit: By Harmid (Own work) [Public domain], via Wikimedia Commons.

A clamped umbilical cord that has been left to pulsate for 3 minutes. Credit: Copyrighted free use, https://commons.wikimedia.org/w/index.php?curid=1428596.

Fathers can have skin-to-skin with the baby if the mother needs medical attention. Credit: Eleanor Hayes.

Chapter 22

Oral Vitamin K is administered. Credit: Ben Barber, USAID, http://www.pixnio.com/science/medical-science/doctor-gives-oral-vaccination-to-an-infant-in-clinic.

References

1 Roser, M., 'Maternal Mortality'. *OurWorldInData.org,* https://ourworldindata.org/maternal-mortality/, 2016

2 Roser, M., 'Child Mortality' *OurWorldInData.org.* https://ourworldindata.org/child-mortality/, 2017

3 'A natural process? Women, men and the medicalisation of childbirth', Science Museum: Bought to Life, http://www.sciencemuseum.org.uk/broughttolife/themes/birthanddeath/childbirthandmedicine

4 Balaskas, J. *Active Birth Centre,* http://activebirthcentre.com/what-is-active-birth/

5 Mongan, M., *Hypnobirthing®: The Mongan Method,* http://www.hypnobirthing-uk.com/

6 Reed, R., 'The assessment of progress', *AIMS* Journal, (2011, vol. 23, no. 2) https://midwifethinking.com/2011/09/14/the-assessment-of-progress/

7 'Birth Choice UK Professional', http://www.birthchoiceuk.com/Professionals/index.html

8 'NHS Maternity Statistics – England, 2016-17', *NHS Digital,* https://digital.nhs.uk/catalogue/PUB30137, 2017

9 Walsh, D., 'Pain and epidural use in normal childbirth', *Evidence Based Midwifery,* Royal College of Midwives, https://www.rcm.org.uk/learning-and-career/learning-and-research/ebm-articles/pain-and-epidural-use-in-normal-childbirth, 2009

10 'Induction of labour: factors to consider', National Institute for Health and Care Excellence, https://pathways.nice.org.uk/pathways/induction-of-labour#path=view%3A/pathways/induction-of-labour/induction-of-labour-factors-to-consider.xmlandcontent=view-node%3Anodes-uncomplicated-pregnancy, 2008.

11 Nolan, M., 'Is this "'evidence"' or a "'best guess'"?', *International Journal of Birth and Parent Education,* http://www.ijbpe.co.uk/index.php/editors-blog/355-is-this-evidence-or-a-best-guess, 2016.

12 England, P., 'Pam England'. *Birthing From Within,* http://www.birthingfromwithin.com/pages/pam-england

13 National Collaborating Centre for Women's and Children's Health, 'Induction of labour', RCOG Press, https://www.nice.org.uk/guidance/cg70/evidence/full-guideline-241871149, 2008.

14 Lothain, J., 'Saying 'No' to Induction', Journal of Perinatal Education, 15(2), 43–45(3) https://www.ncbi.nlm.nih.gov/pmc/articles/PMC1595289/ , 2006

15 Lavender, T., Hart, A., Walkinshaw, S., Campbell, E. and Alfirevic, Z. , 'Progress of first stage of labour for multiparous women: an observational study', BJOG: An International Journal of Obstetrics and Gynaecology, 112: 1663–1665. doi:10.1111/j.1471-0528.2005.00758.x, http://onlinelibrary.wiley.com/doi/10.1111/j.1471-0528.2005.00758.x/abstract, 2005.

16 White, H., Munro, J., and Jokinen, M., 'Evidence based guidelines for midwifery-led care in labour: Latent phase', Royal College of Midwives, https://www.rcm.org.uk/sites/default/files/Latent%20Phase_1.pdf, 2012.

17 Neal, J.L., Lowe, N.K., Ahijevych, K.L., Patrick, T.E., Cabbage, L.A., and Corwin, E.J., "Active labor duration and dilation rates among low-risk, nulliparous women with spontaneous labor onset: a systematic review', *Journal of Midwifery and Women's Health*, Volume 55, Issue 4, http://www.sciencedirect.com/science/article/pii/S1526952309002724, July–August 2010.

18 'Ferguson Reflex', Wikipedia, https://en.wikipedia.org/wiki/Ferguson_reflex, 2017

19 Munro, J., and Jokinen, M., 'Evidence based guidelines for midwifery-led care in labour: second stage of labour', Royal College of Midwives,

https://www.rcm.org.uk/sites/default/files/Second%20Stage%20of%20Labour.pdf, 2012.

20 Taebi M., Kalahroudi M.A., Sadat Z., and Saberi F., 'The duration of the third stage of labor and related factors'. *Iranian Journal of Nursing and Midwifery Research*, 17(2 Suppl 1): S76–S79, https://www.ncbi.nlm.nih.gov/pmc/articles/PMC3696975/, 2012.

21 Pappas, S., 'Yes! Orgasms during birth are real, study suggests', *Livescience*,

http://www.livescience.com/37039-orgasmic-birth-real.html, 2013.

22 Winter, J., 'Hospital Episode Statistics: NHS Maternity Statistics – England, 2013–14', *Hospital Episode Statistics Analysis, Health and Social Care Information Centre*, http://content. digital.nhs.uk/catalogue/PUB16725/nhs-mate-eng-2013-14-summ-repo-rep.pdf, 2015

23 Iladi, P., 'Can -endorphin affect the oxytocin secretion of the brain? A literature review', *Review of Clinical Pharmacology and Pharmacokinetics, International Edition* 22(1): 53–59, January 2008, https://www.researchgate.net/publication/288409292_Can_b-endorphin_affect_the_oxytocin_secretion_of_the_brain_A_literature_review , 2008

24 'Transcutaneous electrical nerve stimulation', Wikipedia, https://en.wikipedia.org/wiki/ Transcutaneous_electrical_nerve_stimulation

25 Dowswell, T., Bedwell, C., Lavender, T., and Neilson, J.P., 'Transcutaneous electrical nerve stimulation (TENS) for pain management in labour'. *Cochrane Database of Systematic Reviews* 2009, Issue 2. Art. No.: CD007214. DOI: 10.1002/14651858.CD007214.pub2. http:// onlinelibrary.wiley.com/doi/10.1002/14651858.CD007214.pub2/abstract, 2009.

26 Bedwell, C., Dowswell, T., Neilson, J.P., and Lavender, T., 'The use of transcutaneous electrical nerve stimulation (TENS) for pain relief in labour: a review of the evidence', *Midwifery*, 27(5), e141 – e148, http://www.midwiferyjournal.com/article/S0266-6138(09)00157-0/abstract, 2011.

27 Robertson, A., 'TENS – A Marketing triumph', Birth International, https://www.birthinternational.com/article/birth/1447/, 2016.

28 'Entonox: The Essential Guide', BOC Healthcare, http://www.bochealthcare.co.uk/internet.lh.lh.gbr/en/images/entonox_essential_guide_hlc401955_Sep10409_64836.pdf

29 'Nitrous oxide (medication)', Wikipedia, https://en.wikipedia.org/wiki/ Nitrous_oxide_(medication)

30 Agah, J., Baghani, R., Hossein, S., Tali, S., and Tabarraei, Y., 'Effects of continuous use of Entonox in comparison with intermittent method on obstetric outcomes: A randomized clinical trial,' *Journal of Pregnancy*, vol. 2014, Article ID 245907, 5 pages, 2014. doi:10.1155/2014/245907, https://www.hindawi.com/journals/jp/2014/245907/, 2014

31 'Entonox', *Anaesthesia* UK, http://www.frca.co.uk/article.aspx?articleid=100364, 2009

32 Hotelling, B. A., 'From psychoprophylactic to orgasmic birth', *The Journal of Perinatal Education*, 18(4), 45–48. http://doi.org/10.1624/105812409X474708

https://www.ncbi.nlm.nih.gov/pmc/articles/PMC2776526/, 2009.

33 Royal College of Midwives, 'How to… administer Entonox', *Midwives magazine*: Issue 2, https://www.rcm.org.uk/news-views-and-analysis/analysis/how-to%E2%80%A6-administer-entonox, 2011.

34 Saxena, K.N., Nischal, H., and Batra, S., 'Intracutaneous injections of sterile water over the secrum for labour analgesia', *Indian Journal of Anaesthesia*, 53(2), 169–173, https://www.ncbi.nlm.nih.gov/pmc/articles/PMC2900101/, 2009.

35 Märtensson, L., McSwiggin, M., and Mercer, J. S., 'US midwives' knowledge and use of sterile water injections for labor pain', *Journal of Midwifery and Women's Health*, 53(2), 115-122. http://www.medscape.com/viewarticle/571287_2, 2008.

36 Simkin, P., and Bolding, A., 'Update on nonpharmacologic approaches to relieve labor pain and prevent suffering', *Journal of Midwifery and Women's Health*, 49(6), http://www.medscape.com/viewarticle/494120_5, 2004.

37 Robinson, J., 'Research. Roundout: pain relief from water Injections', *AIMS Journal*, 11(2), http://www.aims.org.uk/Journal/Vol11No2/ressum99.htm, 1999.

38 Wickham, S., 'Sterile water blocks: Is it time to talk?' *Practising Midwife*, 12(1), 43, http://www.sarawickham.com/wp-content/uploads/2011/10/TPM75-Sterile-water-blocks.pdf, 2009.

39 Derry, S., Straube, S., Moore, R.A., Hancock, H., and Collins, S.L., 'Intracutaneous or subcutaneous sterile water injection compared with blinded controls for pain management in labour', *Cochrane Database of Systematic Reviews* 2012, Issue 1. Art. No.: CD009107. DOI: 10.1002/14651858.CD009107.pub2, http://www.cochrane.org/CD009107/PREG_sterile-water-injections-for-the-relief-of-pain-in-labour, 2012.

40 'Heroin', Wikipedia, https://en.wikipedia.org/wiki/Heroin

41 'Pethidine', Wikipedia, https://en.wikipedia.org/wiki/Pethidine

42 Watts, R. W., 'Does pethidine still have a place in the management of labour pain?', *Australian Prescriber*, Vol 27, No 2., https://www.nps.org.au/australian-prescriber/articles/does-pethidine-still-have-a-place-in-the-management-of-labour-pain#4, 2004

43 'Pain Relief in labour', *NCT*, https://www.nct.org.uk/birth/pain-relief-during-labour#Pethidine

44 'Intrapartum care for healthy women and babies: Clinical guideline [CG190]', *NICE*, https://www.nice.org.uk/guidance/cg190/ifp/chapter/pain-relief, 2017

45 Concordia International, 'Pethidine Injection BP 50mg/ml', *emc+*, https://www.medicines.org.uk/emc/medicine/22031, 2014

46 Lawrence Beech, B., 'Does medication administered to a woman in labour affect the unborn child?', *Association for Improvements in the Maternity Services*, http://www.aims.org.uk/effectDrugsOnBabies.htm, 2014

47 Phillips, S., 'Epidurals: Fact vs. fiction: Do they cause C-sections? Will they harm the baby? Answers to your questions about this popular labor-pain reliever', *Fit Pregnancy and Baby*, http://www.fitpregnancy.com/pregnancy/labor-delivery/epidurals-fact-vs-fiction-0

48 'Epidural Administration', *Wikipedia*, https://en.wikipedia.org/wiki/Epidural_administration

49 'Using epidural anesthesia during labor: Benefits and risks', *American Pregnancy and Labour Association*, http://americanpregnancy.org/labor-and-birth/epidural/, 2017.

50 Bowers, M., 'The truth about walking epidurals: The different kinds of pain relievers, and which one is right for you during labor', *Parenting*, http://www.parenting.com/article/the-truth-about-walking-epidurals, 2017.

51 'Talk: What can you tell me about mobile epidurals?', *Mumsnet*, http://www.mumsnet.com/Talk/childbirth/478238-what-can-you-tell-me-about-mobile-epidurals, 2008

52 Vincent, R.D., and Chestnut, D.H, 'Epidural Analgesia During Labor', *American Family Physician*, Nov 15;58(8):1785-1792, http://www.aafp.org/afp/1998/1115/p1785.html, 1998

53 Silva, M., and Halpern, S. H., 'Epidural analgesia for labor: Current techniques', *Local and Regional Anesthesia*, 3, 143–153. http://doi.org/10.2147/LRA.S10237, https://www.ncbi.nlm.nih.gov/pmc/articles/PMC3417963/, 2010

54 'Epidural', *NHS Choices*, http://www.nhs.uk/Conditions/Epidural-anaesthesia/Pages/Whatitisusedfor.aspx, 2017.

55 MacMillan, A., 'How an epidural may lower postpartum depression risk', *Time Health*, http://time.com/4548397/how-an-epidural-may-lower-postpartum-depression-risk/, 2016

56 Hidaka, R., and Callister, L.C., 'Giving Birth With Epidural Analgesia: The Experience of First-Time Mother, *The Journal of Perinatal Education*, 21(1), 24–35, http://doi.org/10.1891/1058-1243.21.1.24, https://www.ncbi.nlm.nih.gov/pmc/articles/PMC3404542/, 2012.

57 Institute for Quality and Efficiency in Health Care, 'Pregnancy and birth: Epidurals and painkillers for labor pain relief', *PubMed Health*, https://www.ncbi.nlm.nih.gov/pubmed-health/PMH0072751/, 2012.

58 'Epidural risks and side effects', NHS Choices, http://www.nhs.uk/Conditions/Epidural-anaesthesia/Pages/Sideeffects.aspx, 2017

59 Grigg, L., and Day, R., 'Using remifentanil in labour via patient-controlled analgesia', *Nursing Times*, https://www.nursingtimes.net/using-remifentanil-in-labour-via-patient-controlled-analgesia/199872.article, 2003.

60 Buckley, S., 'Epidurals: Risks and concerns for mother and baby', *Sarah Buckley Medical Doctor*, http://sarahbuckley.com/epidurals-risks-and-concerns-for-mother-and-baby, 2009.

61 Anim-Somuah, M., Smyth, R.M.D., and Jones, L., 'Epidural versus non-epidural or no analgesia in labour', *Cochrane Database of Systematic Reviews*, Issue 12. Art. No.: CD000331. DOI: 10.1002/14651858.CD000331.pub3., http://onlinelibrary.wiley.com/doi/10.1002/14651858.CD000331.pub3/abstract, 2011.

62 Anim-Somuah, M., Smyth, R.M.D., and Jones, L., 'Epidurals for pain relief in Labour', Cochrane, http://www.cochrane.org/CD000331/PREG_epidurals-for-pain-relief-in-labour, 2011

63 Baumgarder, D.J., Muehl, P., Fischer, M., and Pribbenow, B., 'Effect of labor epidural anesthesia on breast-feeding of healthy full-term newborns delivered vaginally', *Journal of the American Board of Family Medicine*, 2003, 16(1), http://www.medscape.com/viewarticle/449424, 2003

64 Tussey, C.M., Botsios, E., Gerkin, R.D., Kelly, L.A., Gamez, J., and Mensik, J., 'Reducing length of labor and cesarean surgery rate using a peanut ball for women laboring with an epidural', *The Journal of Perinatal Education*, 24(1), 16–24. http://doi.org/10.1891/1058-1243.24.1.16, https://www.ncbi.nlm.nih.gov/pmc/articles/PMC4748987/, 2012.

65 'What you need to know about: Electronic Foetal Monitoring (CTG)', AIMS Ireland, http://aimsireland.ie/what-you-need-to-know-about-electronic-foetal-monitoring-ctg-2/, 2014.

66 'Fetal heart rate monitoring during labor', *The American College of Obstetricians and Gynecologists*, http://www.acog.org/Patients/FAQs/Fetal-Heart-Rate-Monitoring-During-Labor, 2011.

67 'Fetal scalp blood testing', *Wikipedia*, https://en.wikipedia.org/wiki/Fetal_scalp_blood_testing

68 'External and internal heart rate monitoring of the fetus', *University of Rochester Medical Center Health Encyclopedia*, https://www.urmc.rochester.edu/encyclopedia/content.aspx?contenttypeid=92andcontentid=P07776

69 'Intrapartum care for healthy women and babies: Clinical guideline [CG190]', *National Institute for Health and Clinical Excellence*, https://www.nice.org.uk/guidance/cg190/chapter/recommendations#monitoring-during-labour, 2017.

70 Alfirevic. Z., Devane, D., Gyte, G.M.L., and Cuthbert, A., 'Continuous cardiotocography (CTG) as a form of electronic fetal monitoring (EFM) for fetal assessment during labour', *Cochrane Library*, http://www.cochrane.org/CD006066/PREG_comparing-continuous-electronic-fetal-monitoring-in-labour-cardiotocography-ctg-with-intermittent-listening-intermittent-auscultation-ia, 2017.

71 Dekker, R., 'Evidence-Based Fetal Monitoring', Evidence-Based Birth, http://evidencebasedbirth.com/evidence-based-fetal-monitoring/, 2012.

72 Kavanagh, S., and Payne, J., 'Intrapartum Fetal Monitoring', *Patient*, http://patient.info/

doctor/intrapartum-fetal-monitoring, 2015.

73 Harris, J., 'How to… perform a vaginal examination', Issue 3, *Midwives magazine*, https://www.rcm.org.uk/news-views-and-analysis/analysis/how-to%E2%80%A6-perform-a-vaginal-examination, 2011.

74 'Intrapartum care for healthy women and babies: Clinical guideline [CG190]', *National Institute for Health and Clinical Excellence*, https://www.nice.org.uk/guidance/cg190/chapter/recommendations#monitoring-during-labour, 2017.

75 Munro, J., 'Evidence based guidelines for midwifery-led care in labour: Assessing progress in labour', *Royal College of Midwives*, https://www.rcm.org.uk/sites/default/files/Assessing%20Progress%20in%20%20Labour.pdf, 2012.

76 Derrick, D.C., 'VEs – Essential diagnostic tool?', *AIMS Journal*, 22(2), http://www.aims.org.uk/Journal/Vol22No1/VEsDiagnostic.htm, 2010.

77 Downe, S., Gyte, G.M.L., Dahlen, H.G., and Singata, M., 'Routine vaginal examinations in labour', *Cochrane Library*, http://www.cochrane.org/CD010088/routine-vaginal-examinations-in-labour, 2013.

78 Deckker, R., 'What is the evidence for inducing labor if your water breaks at term?', *Evidence-Based Birth*, http://evidencebasedbirth.com/evidence-inducing-labor-water-breaks-term/, 2014.

79 Shepherd, A., Cheyne, H., Kennedy, S., McIntosh, C., Styles, M., and Niven, C., 'The purple line as a measure of labour progress: A longitudinal study', *BMC Pregnancy and Childbirth*, http://bmcpregnancychildbirth.biomedcentral.com/articles/10.1186/1471-2393-10-54, 2010.

80 'Are vaginal exams accurate?', *Whole Woman*, http://wholewoman.com.au/birth/are-vaginal-exams-accurate, 2015.

81 '5 very good reasons to refuse vaginal exams in labour', *Whole Woman*, http://wholewoman.com.au/birth/vaginal-exams-in-labour-are-not-compulsory, 2016.

82 Reed, R., 'Vaginal examinations: A symptom of a cervical-centric birth culture'. *Midwife Thinking*, https://midwifethinking.com/2015/05/02/vaginal-examinations-a-symptom-of-a-cervix-centric-birth-culture/, 2015.

83 Wickham, S., and Sutton, J., 'The Rhombus of Michaelis: A key to normal birth, or the poor cousin of the RCT?', *Practising Midwife*, 5(11), 22–23, http://sarawickham.com/wp-content/uploads/2011/10/tpm8-the-rhombus-of-michaelis.pdf, 2002.

84 'Bishop Score', *Wikipedia*, https://en.wikipedia.org/wiki/Bishop_score

85 Chamberlain, G., and Zander, L., 'Induction', *BMJ : British Medical Journal*, 318(7189), 995–998, https://www.ncbi.nlm.nih.gov/pmc/articles/PMC1115422/, 1999.

86 Vrouenraets, F.P., Roumen, F.J., Dehing, C.J., van den Akker, E.S., Aarts, M.J., and Scheve, E.J., 'Bishop score and risk of cesarean delivery after induction of labor in nulliparous women', *Obstetric Gynecology*, Apr, 105(4), 690–697, https://www.ncbi.nlm.nih.gov/pubmed/15802392, 2005.

87 Hendrix, N.W., Chauhan, S.P., Morrison, J.C., Magann, E.F., Martin, J.N., and Devoe, L.D., 'Bishop score: A poor diagnostic test to predict failed induction versus vaginal delivery', *South Medical Journal*, Mar, 91(3), 248–252, https://www.ncbi.nlm.nih.gov/pubmed/9521363, 1998.

88 Dekker, R., 'What is the evidence for inducing labor if your water breaks at term?', *Evidence-Based Birth*, http://evidencebasedbirth.com/evidence-inducing-labor-water-breaks-term/, 2014.

89 'Induction of labour', *Gestational Diabetes UK*, http://www.gestationaldiabetes.co.uk/induction/

90 Friberg, A.K., Zingmark, V., and Lyndrup, J., 'Intrahepatic cholestasis of pregnancy: what are the costs?', *Archives of Gynecology and Obstetrics*, October 2016, 294(4), 709–714, https://www.ncbi.nlm.nih.gov/pubmed/26825731

91 Vulliemoz, N.R., and Kurinczuk, J., 'In Vitro Fertilisation: Perinatal risks and early

childhood outcomes', *Royal College of Obstetricians and Gynaecologists,* https://www.rcog.org. uk/globalassets/documents/guidelines/scientific-impact-papers/sip_8.pdf, 2012.

92 'Induction of labour: Evidence tables', *Royal College of Obstetricians and Gynaecologists,* https://www.nice.org.uk/guidance/cg70/evidence/evidence-tables-241871150, 2008.

93 Ewers, H., 'Early induction and shoulder dystocia', *Royal College of Midwives,* https:// www.rcm.org.uk/news-views-and-analysis/news/early-induction-and-shoulder-dystocia, 2015.

94 Whitworth, M.K., Fisher, M., and Heazell, A., 'Reduced fetal movements: Green-top Guideline No. 57', *Royal College of Obstetricians and Gynaecologists,*

https://www.rcog.org.uk/globalassets/documents/guidelines/gtg_57.pdf, 2011.

95 Dekker, R., 'What is the evidence for induction for low amniotic fluid in a healthy pregnancy?', *Science and Sensibility,* https://www.scienceandsensibility.org/p/bl/et/blogid=2andblogaid=503, 2012.

96 Out, J.J., Vierhout, M.E., Verhage, F., Duivenvoorden, H.J., and Wallenburg, H.C., 'Elective induction of labor: A prospective clinical study, II: Psychological effects', *Journal of Perinatal Medicine,* 13(4),163–170., https://www.ncbi.nlm.nih.gov/pubmed/4057032, 1985.

97 'Study Finds Adverse Effects of Pitocin in Newborns', *American College of Obstetricians and Gynecologists,* http://www.acog.org/About-ACOG/News-Room/News-Releases/2013/Study-Finds-Adverse-Effects-of-Pitocin-in-Newborns, 2013.

98 Lothian, J.A., 'Saying "No" to Induction', *Journal of Perinatal Education,* Spring, 15(2), 43–45, PMCID: PMC1595289, https://www.ncbi.nlm.nih.gov/pmc/articles/PMC1595289/, 2006.

99 UT Southwestern Medical Center, 'Molecular mechanisms within fetal lungs initiate labor', *ScienceDaily,* www.sciencedaily.com/releases/2015/06/150622162023.htm, 2015.

100 Hayes, E., 'I'm a baby, get me out of here: Natural ways to induce labour', Birthzang, *http://www.birthzang.co.uk/2013/11/start-labour-naturally/,* 2013.

101 National Collaborating Centre for Women's and Children's Health (UK), 'Induction of Labour: 7, Monitoring and pain relief for induction of labour (NICE Clinical Guidelines, No. 70.)', *RCOG Press,* https://www.ncbi.nlm.nih.gov/books/NBK53623/, 2008.

102 Stock, S.J., Ferguson, E., Duffy, A., Ford, I., Chalmers, J., Norman, J.E., et al., 'Outcomes of elective induction of labour compared with expectant management: Population based study', *BMJ,* 344 :e2838, http://www.bmj.com/content/344/bmj.e2838, 2012.

103 Gibbon, K., 'How to... perform a stretch and sweep',
Midwives Magazine, Issue 1, https://www.rcm.org.uk/news-views-and-analysis/analysis/how-to%E2%80%80%A6-perform-a-stretch-and-sweep, 2012.

104 McCulloch, S., 'Membrane sweep – 6 facts to consider before having one', *BellyBelly.au,* http://www.bellybelly.com.au/birth/membrane-sweep-6-facts/, 2016.

105 Katakam, N., Muotune, C.A., Tomlinson, A.J., and Chia, K.V., 'Guideline for induction of labour – Propess, cervical ripening balloon, Prostaglandin gel', *Bolton NHS Foundation Trust,* http://www.boltonft.nhs.uk/wp-content/uploads/2013/05/Induction-of-Labour-Guideline-17-1-13-amended-JT-NK.pdf, 2011.

106 Boulvain, M., Stan, C.M., and Irion, O., 'Membrane sweeping for induction of labour', *Cochrane Library,* http://www.cochrane.org/CD000451/PREG_membrane-sweeping-for-induction-of-labour, 2002.

107 Lemay, G., 'Membrane stripping, membrane sweeping–just say NO', *Wise Woman Way of Birth,* http://wisewomanwayofbirth.com/membrane-stripping-membrane-sweeping-just-say-no/, 2016.

108 Zamzami, T., and Al Senani, N., 'The efficacy of membrane sweeping at term and effect on the duration of pregnancy: A randomized controlled trial', *Journal Of Clinical Gynecology And Obstetrics,* 3(1), 30–34, http://www.jcgo.org/index.php/jcgo/article/view/225/97, 2014.

109 Boulvain, M., Stan, C., and Irion, O., 'Membrane sweeping for induction of labour', *Cochrane Database of Systematic Reviews*, https://www.ncbi.nlm.nih.gov/pubmed/11405964, 2001.

110 'Prostaglandin E2', *Wikipedia*, https://en.wikipedia.org/wiki/Prostaglandin_E2

111 Thomas, J., Fairclough, A., Kavanagh, J., and Kelly, A.J., 'Vaginal prostaglandin (PGE2 and PGF2a) for induction of labour at term', *Cochrane Library*, http://www.cochrane.org/CD003101/PREG_vaginal-prostaglandin-pge2-and-pgf2a-for-induction-of-labour-at-term, 2014.

112 'PROPESS® 10 mg vaginal delivery system: dinoprostone', *EMC*, http://www.medicines.org.uk/emc/PIL.18005.latest.pdf, 2016.

113 'Prostin E2 Vaginal Tablets', *EMC*, https://www.medicines.org.uk/emc/medicine/1563, 2014.

114 Kalkat, R.K., McMillan, E., Cooper, H., and Palmer, K., 'Comparison of Dinoprostone slow release pessary (Propess) with gel (Prostin) for induction of labour at term: A randomised trial', *Journal of Obstetrics and Gynaecology*, 28(7): 695–699, http://www.crd.york.ac.uk/crdweb/ShowRecord.asp?LinkFrom=OAIandID=2200910023, 2008.

115 Thomas, J., Fairclough, A., Kavanagh, J., and Kelly, A.J., 'Vaginal prostaglandin (PGE2 and PGF2a) for induction of labour at term', *Cochrane Database of Systematic Reviews*, Issue 6. Art. No.: CD003101. DOI: 10.1002/14651858.CD003101.pub3. https://www.ncbi.nlm.nih.gov/pubmedhealth/PMH0011817/, 2014.

116 'Foley Catheter', Wikipedia, https://en.wikipedia.org/wiki/Foley_catheter

117 Yates, J., 'New data: Foley catheter is as effective as prostaglandin gel for induction of labor—with fewer side effects', *OBG Management*, November, 23(11), http://www.mdedge.com/obgmanagement/article/64539/obstetrics/new-data-foley-catheter-effective-prostaglandin-gel-induction, 2011.

118 'Prostaglandin induction and vaginal delivery rates (query bank), *Royal College of Obstetricians and Gynaecologists*, https://www.rcog.org.uk/en/guidelines-research-services/guidelines/prostaglandin-induction-and-vaginal-delivery-rates---query-bank/, 2014.

119 'Artificial Rupture of Membranes', Wikipedia, https://en.wikipedia.org/wiki/Artificial_rupture_of_membranes

120 O'Connell, N.G., 'Amniotomy: background', Medscape, http://emedicine.medscape.com/article/1997932-overview?pa=ekuyl0ihVtRlScRjsTRM82R%2B91cg-J%2FNPT9SGCdCDObH5wnZbaph0Fs8HHdJlwqEqY8KH7JRRTLCwxPErpBxJilaycSibeA-0Q%2FJsWK%2BpGHzs%3D#a6, 2016.

121 Munro, J., and Jokinen, M., 'Evidence based guidelines for midwifery-led care in labour: Rupturing membranes', *Royal College of Midwives*, https://www.rcm.org.uk/sites/default/files/Rupturing%20Membranes.pdf, 2012

122 Fraser, W.D., Turcot, L., Krauss, I., and Brisson-Carrol, G. 'Amniotomy for shortening spontaneous labour', *Cochrane Database Systematic Review*, 2):CD000015. https://www.ncbi.nlm.nih.gov/pubmed/10796086, 2002.

123 Fraser, W.D., Marcoux, S., Moutquin, J-M., Christen, A., et al., 'Effect of early amniotomy on the risk of dystocia in nulliparous women', *New England Journal of Medicine*, 328(16), http://www.nejm.org/doi/pdf/10.1056/NEJM199304223281602, 1993.

124 Sloame Cohain, J., 'Amniotomy and cord prolapse', *Midwifery today with international midwife*, https://www.researchgate.net/publication/260150939_Amniotomy_and_cord_prolapse, 2013.

125 Vincent, M., 'Amniotomy: to do or not to do?', *Midwives Magazine*, https://www.rcm.org.uk/news-views-and-analysis/analysis/amniotomy-to-do-or-not-to-do, 2005.

126 Brusie, C., 'Pitocin Induction: The Risks and Benefits', *Healthline*, http://www.healthline.com/health/pregnancy/pitocin-induction#Overview1, 2016

127 'Syntocinon', *Sandoz Pharmaceuticals Corporation*, https://www.drugs.com/pro/

syntocinon.html, 2006

128 'Induction', Wikipedia, https://en.wikipedia.org/wiki/Labor_induction

129 'Inducing Labour', NHS Choices, http://www.nhs.uk/conditions/pregnancy-and-ba-by/pages/induction-labour.aspx, 2017

130 Alfirevic, Z., Baxter, J., Calder, A., Green, J., Markham, C., McCormick, C., Shehata, H., Smales Hill, S., Stewart, M., Stewart, P., Tubman, R., 'NICE Clinical Guideline 70 – Induction of Labour', http://www.nhs.uk/planners/pregnancycareplanner/documents/nice_induc-tion_of_labour.pdf, 2008

131 'Compare Medicines: Pitocin vs Syntocinon', Treato, https://treato.com/Pitocin,Syntocinon/?a=s

132 Cunha, J.P., 'Pitocin side effects center', RxList, http://www.rxlist.com/pitocin-side-ef-fects-drug-center.htm, 2016.

133 'Pitocin side effects', Drugs.com, https://www.drugs.com/sfx/pitocin-side-effects.html

134 'Syntocinon', Drugs.com, https://www.drugs.com/pro/syntocinon.html, 1996.

135 'Study finds adverse effects of Pitocin in newborns', The American College of Obstetri-cians and Gynecologists, http://www.acog.org/About-ACOG/News-Room/News-Releas-es/2013/Study-Finds-Adverse-Effects-of-Pitocin-in-Newborns, 2013.

136 'Inducing Labour (NICE Clinical Guideline CG70)', National Institute for Health and Clinical Excellence (UK), https://www.nice.org.uk/guidance/CG70/chapter/1-Guid-ance#prevention-and-management-of-complications, 2008.

137 Axman, L., 'Pitocin's untold impact', Birthfaith, http://birthfaith.org/pitocin/pito-cins-untold-impact, 2010.

138 Bell, A.F., Erickson, E.N., and Carter, C.S., 'Beyond labor: The role of natural and synthet-ic oxytocin in the transition to motherhood', Journal of Midwifery and Women's Health, 59(1), 35–42. http://doi.org/10.1111/jmwh.12101, https://www.ncbi.nlm.nih.gov/pmc/articles/PMC3947469/, 2014

139 'Ergometrine', Wikipdia, https://en.wikipedia.org/wiki/ergometrine

140 'Syntometrine Ampoules', EMC, https://www.medicines.org.uk/emc/medicine/135, 2016.

141 'Postpartum haemorrhage: Ergometrine (query bank)', Royal College of Obstetricians and Gynaecologists, https://www.rcog.org.uk/en/guidelines-research-services/guide-lines/postpartum-haemorrhage-ergometrine---query-bank/, 2013.

142 Baker, K., 'How to... manage primary postpartum haemorrhage', Midwives magazine, Issue 4, https://www.rcm.org.uk/news-views-and-analysis/analysis/how-to-manage-pri-mary-postpartum-harmorrhage, 2014

143 RCOG Patient Information Committee, 'Information for you Heavy bleeding after birth (postpartum haemorrhage)', Royal College of Obstetricians and gynaecologists, https://www.rcog.org.uk/globalassets/documents/patients/patient-information-leaflets/pregnan-cy/heavy-bleeding-after-birth.pdf, 2013.

144 Baker, K., How to... conduct active management of the third stage of labour', Midwives magazine, Issue 6, https://www.rcm.org.uk/news-views-and-analysis/analysis/how-to-conduct-active-management-of-the-third-stage-of-labour, 2013.

145 'What you should know about Syntometrine®', Sandoz Pharmaceuticals, http://mcs.open.ac.uk/nlg/old_projects/pills/corpus/pil/data/Sandoz/Syntometrine/Syntometrine.html, 1995.

146 National Collaborating Centre for Women's and Children's Health (UK), 'Intrapartum care: Care of healthy women and their babies during childbirth: 13, Third stage of labour (NICE Clinical Guidelines, No. 190.)', National Institute for Health and Care Excellence (UK); https://www.ncbi.nlm.nih.gov/books/NBK328242/, 2014

147 Begley, C.M., Gyte, G.M., Devane, D., McGuire, W., and Weeks, A., 'Active versus expect-ant management for women in the third stage of labour', The Cochrane Database of Systematic

Reviews, (11), CD007412, http://doi.org/10.1002/14651858.CD007412.pub3, 2011.

148 White, H., Munro, J., and Jokinen, M., 'Evidence based guidelines for midwifery-led care in labour: Third stage of labour, Royal College of Midwives, https://www.rcm.org.uk/sites/default/files/Third%20Stage%20of%20Labour.pdf, 2012.

149 Begley, C.M., Gyte, G.M.L., Devane, D., McGuire, W., and Weeks, A., 'Delivering the placenta with active, expectant or mixed management in the third stage of labour', *Cochrane Library*, http://www.cochrane.org/CD007412/PREG_delivering-the-placenta-with-active-expectant-or-mixed-management-in-the-third-stage-of-labour, 2015.

150 Begley, C.M., Gyte, G.M.L., Devane, D., McGuire, W., and Weeks, A., 'Active versus expectant management for women in the third stage of labour', *Cochrane Database of Systematic Reviews*, https://www.ncbi.nlm.nih.gov/pubmed/22071837, 2015.

151 'Episiotomy', Wikipedia, https://en.wikipedia.org/wiki/Episiotomy

152 Gibbon, K., 'How to perform an episiotomy', *Midwives magazine*, Issue 5, https://www.rcm.org.uk/news-views-and-analysis/analysis/how-to-perform-an-episiotomy, 2012.

153 Bick, D., Munro, J., and Jokinen, M., 'Evidence Based Guidelines for Midwifery-Led Care in Labour: Care of the Perineum', Royal College of Midwives, https://www.rcm.org.uk/sites/default/files/Care%20of%20the%20Perineum.pdf, 2012.

154 'Episiotomy or tear during childbirth', NCT, https://www.nct.org.uk/parenting/episiotomy-or-tear-during-childbirth

155 'NHS Maternity Statistics – England, 2010–2011', *NHS Digital*, http://content.digital.nhs.uk/pubs/maternity1011, 2011.

156 Mullally, A., and Murphy, D.J., 'Episiotomy', *Global Library of Women's Medicine*, *(ISSN: 1756-2228)* 2011; DOI 10.3843/GLOWM.10128, https://www.glowm.com/section_view/heading/Episiotomy/item/128, 2011.

157 Bhattacharjee, R., 'Episiotomy vs perineal tear –A Comparative study of maternal and fetal outcome', *IOSR Journal of Dental and Medical Sciences*,13(11), 8–11, Ver. V (November) e-ISSN: 2279-0853, p-ISSN: 2279-0861. http://www.iosrjournals.org/iosr-jdms/papers/Vol13-issue11/Version-5/B0131150811.pdf, 2014.

158 Lappen, J.R., 'Episiotomy and Repair', Medscape, http://emedicine.medscape.com/article/2047173-overview#a5, 2016.

159 Viswanathan, M., Hartmann, K., Palmieri, R., et al., 'The use of episiotomy in obstetrical care: A systematic review: Summary in AHRQ evidence report summaries', *Agency for Healthcare Research and Quality*, 1998-2005. 112., https://www.ncbi.nlm.nih.gov/books/NBK11967/, 2005.

160 Beckmann, M.M., and Stock, O.M., 'Antenatal perineal massage for reducing perineal trauma', *Cochrane Database of Systematic Reviews*, 2013 Apr 30(4),CD005123. doi: 10.1002/14651858.CD005123.pub3, 2013.
https://www.ncbi.nlm.nih.gov/pubmed/23633325?dopt=Abstract

161 'How to do perineal massage', Wiki How to do Anything, http://www.wikihow.com/Do-Perineal-Massage

162 'Clinical Studies and References', *Epi-No Birth Preparation*, http://www.epino.de/en/studies-epino.html

163 Kok, J., Tan, K.H., Koh, S., Cheng, P.S., Lim, W.Y., Yew, M.L., and Yeo, G.S.,'Antenatal use of a novel vaginal birth training device by term primiparous women in Singapore', *Singapore Medical Journal*, 45(7),318–323., https://www.ncbi.nlm.nih.gov/pubmed/15221047, 2004.

164 Bohatá, P., and Dostálek, L., 'The possibility of antepartal prevention of episiotomy and perineal tears during delivery', *Ceska Gynekologie*, 81(3),192–201. [Article in Czech], https://www.ncbi.nlm.nih.gov/pubmed/27882762, 2016.

165 Aasheim, V., Nilsen, A.B., Lukasse, M., and Reinar, L.M., 'Perineal techniques during the second stage of labour for reducing perineal trauma', *Cochrane Database of Systematic Reviews*, 7;(12):CD006672. doi: 10.1002/14651858.CD006672.pub2., https://www.ncbi.nlm.nih.gov/pubmed/22161407?dopt=Abstract, 2011.

166 Munro, J., and Jokinen, M., 'Evidence based guidelines for midwifery-led care in labour positions for labour and birth', Royal College of Midwives, https://www.rcm.org.uk/sites/default/files/Positions%20for%20Labour%20and%20Birth.pdf, 2012.

167 Gizzo, S., Di Gangi, S., Noventa, M., Bacile, V., Zambon, A., and Battista Nardelli, G., 'Women's choice of positions during labour: Return to the Past or a Modern Way to Give Birth? A cohort study in Italy', BioMed Research International, vol. 2014, Article ID 638093, 7 pages, 2014. doi:10.1155/2014/638093, https://www.hindawi.com/journals/bmri/2014/638093/2014

168 Meyvis, I., Van Rommpaey, B., Goormans, K., Truijen, S., Lambers, S., Mestdagh, E., and Mistiaen, W., 'Maternal position and other variables: effects on perineal outcomes in 557 births', Birth, 39(2),115–120, https://www.researchgate.net/publication/234041654_Maternal_Position_and_Other_Variables_Effects_on_Perineal_Outcomes_in_557_Births, 2012.

169 DiFranco, J.T., and Curl, M., 'Healthy birth practice #5: Avoid giving birth on your back and follow your body's urge to push', The Journal of Perinatal Education, 23(4), 207–210, https://www.ncbi.nlm.nih.gov/pmc/articles/PMC4235063/, 2014.

170 'Labor and delivery, postpartum care: The role of warm compresses and tissue massage', The Mayo Clinic, http://www.mayoclinic.org/healthy-lifestyle/labor-and-delivery/in-depth/episiotomy/art-20047282?pg=2, 2015.

171 'Episiotomy or tear during childbirth', NCT, https://www.nct.org.uk/parenting/episiotomy-or-tear-during-childbirth

172 'Forceps in childbirth', Wikipedia, https://en.wikipedia.org/wiki/Forceps_in_childbirth

173 'ventouse', Wikipedia, https://en.wikipedia.org/wiki/Ventouse

174 Ali, U.A., and Norwitz, E.R., 'Vacuum-assisted vaginal delivery', Reviews in Obstetrics and Gynecology, 2(1), 5–17, https://www.ncbi.nlm.nih.gov/pmc/articles/PMC2672989/, 2009.

175 'Indications for instrumental delivery', StratOG, https://stratog.rcog.org.uk/tutorial/obstetrics/indications-for-instrumental-delivery-5827

176 Garrison, A., 'Vacuum extraction', Medscape, http://emedicine.medscape.com/article/271175-overview#a4

177 Patel, R.R., and Murphy, D.J., 'Forceps delivery in modern obstetric practice', BMJ: British Medical Journal, 328(7451), 1302–1305, https://www.ncbi.nlm.nih.gov/pmc/articles/PMC420176/, 2004.

178 Hafeez, M., Badar, N., and Yasin, A., 'Indications and Risks of Vacuum Assisted Deliveries', Journal International Medical Sciences Academy, October-December Vol. 26 No. 4, 2013. http://medind.nic.in/jav/t13/i4/javt13i4p213.pdf

179 Farrell, S.A., 'Cesarean section versus forceps-assisted vaginal birth: It's time to include pelvic injury in the risk–benefit equation', CMAJ: Canadian Medical Association Journal, 166(3), 337–338, https://www.ncbi.nlm.nih.gov/pmc/articles/PMC99315/, 2002.

180 O'Mahony, F., Hofmeyr, G.J., and Menon, V., 'Instruments for assisted vaginal delivery', Cochrane Library, http://www.cochrane.org/CD005455/PREG_instruments-for-assisted-vaginal-delivery, 2010.

181 Colli, R., Biagiotti, I., and Sterpa, A., 'Osteopathy in neonatology', Medical and surgical paediatrics, Mar-Apr, 25(2):101–105, https://www.ncbi.nlm.nih.gov/pubmed/12916435, 2003.

182 Anim-Somuah, M., Smyth, R.M.D., and Jones, L., 'Epidural versus non-epidural or no analgesia in labour (Review)', Cochrane Database of Systematic Reviews, Issue 12. Art. No.: CD000331. DOI: 10.1002/14651858.CD000331.pub3., http://onlinelibrary.wiley.com/store/10.1002/14651858.CD000331.pub3/asset/CD000331.pdf?v=1andt=j0ntgkemands=1ab074e2fd5219735f8b1c345a0c7ed5cc2b72cf, 2011.

183 Ali, U.A., and Norwitz, E.R. , 'Vacuum-assisted vaginal delivery', Reviews in Obstetrics and Gynecology, 2(1), 5–17, https://www.ncbi.nlm.nih.gov/pmc/articles/PMC2672989/, 2009.

184 Thomas, D.B., 'Aetiological associations in infantile colic: An hypothesis', Journal of Paediatrics and Child Health, 17: 292–295. doi:10.1111/j.1440-1754.1981.tb01963.x, http://

onlinelibrary.wiley.com/doi/10.1111/j.1440-1754.1981.tb01963.x/abstract, 1981.

185 Ockwell-Smith, S., '5 REASONS WHY YOUR BIRTH CAN AFFECT YOUR BABY AND YOUR PARENTING', Sarah Ockwell-Smith, https://sarahockwell-smith.com/2012/11/04/5-reasons-why-your-birth-can-affect-your-baby-and-your-parenting/, 2012.

186 'Caesarean section', Wikipedia, https://en.wikipedia.org/wiki/Caesarean_section

187 Caesarean section, clinical guidance [CG132]', National Institute for Health and Clinical Excellence (NICE), https://www.nice.org.uk/guidance/cg132, 2011.

188 'What happens during elective or emergency C-sections?', NCT, https://www.nct.org.uk/birth/what-happens-during-elective-or-emergency-caesarean-section#operation

189 'Caesarean section', NHS Choices, http://www.nhs.uk/Conditions/Caesarean-section/Pages/Introduction.aspx#why, 2016.

190 'Caesarean birth: What are the risks and benefits?', BabyCentre, http://www.babycentre.co.uk/a1029062/caesarean-birth-what-are-the-risks-and-benefits, 2016

191 'Risks of a caesarean section', NHS Choices, http://www.nhs.uk/Conditions/Caesarean-section/Pages/Risks.aspx, 2016.

192 Olde, E., van der Hart, O., Klebera, R., and van Sona, M., 'Post-traumatic stress following childbirth: A review', Clinical Psychology Review, 26(1), http://www.sciencedirect.com/science/article/pii/S0272735805000991, 2006.

193 Renz-Polster, H., David, M.R., Buist, A.S., Vollmer, W.M., O'Connor, E.A., Frazier, E.A., and Wall, M.A., 'Caesarean section delivery and the risk of allergic disorders in childhood', Clinical and Experimental Allergy, Nov, 35(11),1466–1472. https://www.ncbi.nlm.nih.gov/pubmed/16297144, 2005.

194 'Risks of caesarean section – research papers', AIMS, http://www.aims.org.uk/OccasionalPapers/risksOfCaesareanSections.pdf, 2008.

195 Magee, S.R., Battle, C., Morton, J., and Nothnagle, M.J., 'Promotion of family-centered birth with gentle cesarean delivery', Journal of the American Board of Family Medicine, 27(5), 690–693. doi: 10.3122/jabfm.2014.05.140014. http://www.jabfm.org/content/27/5/690.full, 2014.

196 Meghan, B., Azad, T.K., Maughan, H., Guttman, D.S., Field, C.J., Chari, R.S., Sears, M.R., Becker, A.B., Scott, J.A., and Kozyrskyj, A.L., on behalf of the CHILD Study Investigators, 'Gut microbiota of healthy Canadian infants: Profiles by mode of delivery and infant diet at 4 months' CMAJ, March 19, 185(5) First published February 11, 2013, doi:10.1503/cmaj.121189 http://www.cmaj.ca/content/185/5/385, 2013.

197 Neu, J., and Rushing, J., 'Cesarean versus vaginal delivery: Long term infant outcomes and the Hygiene Hypothesis', Clinics in Perinatology, Jun, 38(2): 321–331. doi: 10.1016/j.clp.2011.03.008 https://www.ncbi.nlm.nih.gov/pmc/articles/PMC3110651/, 2011

198 Microbirth, http://microbirth.com/

199 Domenjoz, I., Kayser, B., and Boulvain, M., 'Effect of physical activity during pregnancy on mode of delivery', American Journal of Obstetrics and Gynecology, Oct, 211(4), 401.e1–11. doi: 10.1016/j.ajog.2014.03.030. Epub 2014 Mar 14. https://www.ncbi.nlm.nih.gov/pubmed/24631706, 2014

200. Hung, K.J., and Berg, O., 'Early skin-to-skin after cesarean to improve breastfeeding', The American Journal of Maternal Child Nursing, Sep-Oct, 36(5), 318–324; quiz 325-6. doi: 10.1097/NMC.0b013e3182266314. https://www.ncbi.nlm.nih.gov/pubmed/21743355, 2011.

201 Pereira Gomes Morais, E., Riera, R., Porfírio, G.J.M., Macedo, C.R., Sarmento Vasconcelos, V., de Souza Pedrosa, A., Torloni, M.R. 'Chewing gum for enhancing early recovery of bowel function after caesarean section', Cochrane Database of Systematic Reviews 2016, Issue 10. Art. No.: CD011562. DOI: 10.1002/14651858.CD011562.pub2. http://www.cochrane.org/CD011562/PREG_does-chewing-gum-after-caesarean-section-lead-quicker-recovery-bowel-function

202 'What is the umbilical cord?', NHS Choices, http://www.nhs.uk/chq/pages/2299.

aspx?categoryid=54, 2005.

203 Crews, C., 'Clamping of the umbilical cord – immediate or delayed – is this really an issue?' Midwifery Services South Texas, http://www.midwiferyservices.org/umbilical_cord_clamping.htm,

204 Burleigh, A., and Tizard, H., 'Latest recommendations on timing of clamping the umbilical cord', Royal College of Midwives, https://www.rcm.org.uk/news-views-and-analysis/views/latest-recommendations-on-timing-of-clamping-the-umbilical-cord, 2015.

205 'RCOG release: Timing of clamping the umbilical cord analysed in new opinion paper', Royal College of Obstetricians and Gynaecologists, https://www.rcog.org.uk/en/news/rcog-release-timing-of-clamping-the-umbilical-cord-analysed-in-new-opinion-paper/, 2015.

206 'Intrapartum care: Quality standard [QS105]', National Institute for Health and Care Excellence (NICE), https://www.nice.org.uk/guidance/qs105/chapter/quality-statement-6-delayed-cord-clamping, 2015.

207 'Optimal timing of cord clamping for the prevention of iron deficiency anaemia in infants', World Health Organization, http://www.who.int/elena/titles/full_recommendations/cord_clamping/en/, 2012.

208 Wyllie, J., Ainsworth, S., and Tinnion, R., 'Resuscitation and support of transition of babies at birth', Resuscitation Council (UK), https://www.resus.org.uk/resuscitation-guidelines/resuscitation-and-support-of-transition-of-babies-at-birth/, 2015.

209 Rabe, H., Diaz-Rossello, J.L., Duley, L., and Dowswell, T., 'Effect of timing of umbilical cord clamping and other strategies to influence placental transfusion at preterm birth on maternal and infant outcomes', Cochrane Database of Systematic Reviews, Issue 8. Art. No.: CD003248. DOI: 10.1002/14651858.CD003248.pub3, https://www.ncbi.nlm.nih.gov/pubmedhealth/PMH0011919/, 2012.

210 Raju, T.N.K., and Singal, N., 'Optimal timing for clamping the umbilical cord after birth', Clinics in Perinatology, 39(4), 10.1016/j.clp.2012.09.006. 2013, https://www.ncbi.nlm.nih.gov/pmc/articles/PMC3835342/, 2012.

211 Bonyata, K., 'Is iron-supplementation necessary?', IBCLC, Kellymom Breastfeeding Parenting http://kellymom.com/nutrition/vitamins/iron/, 2012.

212 Lippi, G., and Franchini, M., 'Vitamin K in neonates: facts and myths', Blood Transfusion, Jan, 9(1): 4–9, National Center for Biotechnology Information https://www.ncbi.nlm.nih.gov/pmc/articles/PMC3021393/, 2011.

213 'Getting to know your newborn', NHS Choices, http://www.nhs.uk/conditions/pregnancy-and-baby/pages/your-baby-after-birth.aspx, 2015.

214 Dekker, R., 'Evidence for the vitamin K shot in newborns', Evidence-Based Birth, https://evidencebasedbirth.com/evidence-for-the-vitamin-k-shot-in-newborns/, 2014.

215 Malik, S., Udani, R.H., Bichile, S.K., Agrawal, R.M., Bahrainwala, A.T., and Tilaye, S., 'Comparative study of oral versus injectable vitamin K in neonates', Indian Pediatric, Jul, 29(7), 857-859. https://www.ncbi.nlm.nih.gov/pubmed/1428134, 1992.

216 'Vitamin K: Injection or oral dose for newborns', NCT, https://www.nct.org.uk/parenting/vitamin-k

217 PANDAS Foundation http://www.pandasfoundation.org.uk/information/

Index

Don't Forget

TO LEAVE A REVIEW
ON AMAZON OR KINDLE

For blog posts to help you enjoy an awesome pregnancy, labour and birth and parenthood go to

www.birthzang.co.uk

Most popular articles:

7 Top Tips to Help Pelvic Pain in Pregnancy

Cooking Times May Vary (by 5 Weeks), or the Curse of the EDD

I'm a Baby! Get Me Out of Here! – Natural Ways to Induce Labour

Birthzang's Guide to using Clary Sage Oil in Labour

DON'T say this to someone who has had a Miscarriage (but say THIS instead)

5 Things Every Parent Should Know About Newborn Babies

How to wind a baby … Birthzang's Amazing Baby Burp Technique!

As the Wind Blows…Birthzang's Amazing Baby Fart Expulsion Technique!

Join our Facebook support group for parents.

www.facebook.com/groups/
BirthzangParentsSupportGroup/

Printed in Poland
by Amazon Fulfillment
Poland Sp. z o.o., Wrocław